Healing your Emotions

Healing your Emotions

Angela Hicks & John Hicks

Thorsons
An Imprint of HarperCollins*Publishers*

Thorsons
An Imprint of HarperCollins*Publishers*
77–85 Fulham Palace Road,
Hammersmith, London W6 8JB
Published by Thorsons 1999
The Thorsons website address is:
www.thorsons.com

978-0-00-732640-2

Text illustrations by Su Eaton

Contents

AUTHORS' NOTE

We have capitalized all Chinese medical terminology in this book in order to differentiate it from standard English terms.

Our thanks to all of the people who have helped us with this book, especially: Mark Allan; Marguerite Beckerlegge; Gill Black; Janice Booth; Heather Bovey; Mark Bovey; Sally Blades; Judith Clark; Tony Connor; Di Cook; Ian Dixon; Di Eckersley; Jane Ford;Julia Funk; Rosemarie Gallagher; Gaby Hock; Sue Horne; Lizzie Hubbard; David James; Mary Kaspar; Chris Kear; Lawerence Kershen; Stella King; Magda Koc; Madelaine Molder; Carey Morgan; Keith Murray; Ilana Pearlman; Barbara Pickett; Fiona Reynoldson; Jane Robinson; Jo Rochford; Sandy Sandaver; Marcus Senior; Kath Simmonds; Deborah Thomson; Carmel Twomey; Penny Wilson; Julie Wisbey.

We would also like to thank all of the people who have come to our 'Oral Tradition' workshops which we set up to deepen understanding of the Five Element types.

All names have been changed for confidentiality.

Secondly, we would also like to thank the people who have taken the time to read through this book and comment on it. Especially Judith Clark, Jane Grossfeld, Sophie Hayes, Gaby Hock, Helen Knotts and Peter Mole.

Thirdly, we would like to thank everyone who contributed to our learning of NLP, especially Eileen Seymour-Watkins, Graham Dawes, Gene Early and Robert Dilts. We would also like to thank Richard Bandler, one of the co-creators of NLP.

Finally, we wish to thank all the people who have enabled us to learn this style of Chinese Medicine. Most of all we wish to thank JR Worsley who originally taught us acupuncture and demonstrated the skills of Five Element diagnosis with such elegance. We would also like to thank all of our friends and colleagues who we worked with at the Oxford Acupuncture Clinic in Farmoor including Judy Becker-Worsley, Meriel Derby, Julia Measures, Peter Mole and Allegra Wint. We learned so much with you over those years. We would also like to thank all those who make the college function so well, including Helen, Wanda, Sean and Julian. Also everyone on the faculty of the College of Integrated Chinese Medicine who by their teaching give support for the development of the acupuncture and herbal medicine professions.

INTRODUCTION

WHY WE WROTE THIS BOOK AND WHAT TO EXPECT FROM IT

Alex, a friend of ours, went to a Chinese doctor for some herbs — she had a number of ailments — digestive problems, headaches and insomnia. The doctor asked her questions about her health then took some minutes to carefully feel the 12 pulses on her wrist — an important part of Chinese Traditional diagnosis.

Finally the doctor sat back, his diagnosis completed. He looked her straight in the eye and told her, 'Your problem is that you worry too much. You must stop worrying.' Alex was — unusually — stunned to silence by the doctor's directness. She merely nodded and said, 'Yes I'll stop worrying'. Later that day as we talked on the phone we all laughed as she started to worry about how to stop worrying!

This book is all about your emotions and your health. It will provide you with many important tools. One of these is to help you to identify the main emotions which repeatedly stop you from becoming healthy. For Alex this was worry. She later recognized that the wise Chinese doctor was very accurate in diagnosing this as the cause of her problems. She then set about discovering how to stop worrying. Do you think Alex could immediately stop worrying? The answer is no, of course she couldn't.

Alex realized very quickly that it is one thing to know that our emotions are adversely affecting our health but quite another to know what to do about it. So the other tool this book will provide is many practical exercises to deal with those emotions so that we can become healthier. We hope the result will be that you feel better in every way — physically, mentally and spiritually.

About This Book

This book brings together two areas of knowledge — one Eastern and one Western. The Eastern one comes from the ancient theory of the Five Elements. The theory of the Five Elements is discussed in greater detail in the first chapter. A system of 'constitutional types' is derived from this theory.

This system of constitutional types describes five types of people. For each type there is a shared set of core beliefs, values and concerns, and ways of expressing ourselves emotionally. By understanding these types we can gain a head start in the process of knowing where to work on ourselves.

The Western area of knowledge comes mainly from Neuro-linguistic Programming. We are both trained as practitioners in this therapy. We also draw from other therapies such as Gestalt and a system called 'Focusing'.

Neuro-linguistic Programming (NLP) has created methods which enable people to work on their deepest mental or emotional processes. These include their beliefs, attitudes, values and patterns of emotional expression. By changing these processes, people can start to experience themselves more positively and constructively. If we *believe*, for instance, that people like to help each other and that, generally, we can learn and grow, we will be more likely to be helped, learn and grow. If, on the other hand, we *believe* people are generally selfish and don't want to help each other and that we are no good at learning and growing, then we are less likely to get help and learn and grow.[1]

As well as the therapies mentioned above we have added Qigong exercises which help the Organs. The Chinese have carefully researched and proved the effectiveness of these exercises for many specific diseases. In fact, Qi Gong exercises are taught in Chinese medical colleges as a method of treatment. As well as including a relevant exercise for each type we will also refer you to sources to find further ones.[2]

This book puts the Five Element constitutional types and therapeutic exercises together. Once we have determined our Five Element constitutional type, we have a pathway to our significant values, attitudes and patterns of emotional expression. Then, using the exercises designed for each constitutional type, we can work on the very structure which creates our world. This will in turn allow us to become more balanced. Ultimately this means smoother, more positive and more enjoyable emotions and, in the end, greater health.

How This Book Came About

As authors, we both have over 20 years of experience as practitioners of Chinese medicine. Chinese medicine teaches that healthy emotions are a natural part of living but also that certain types of emotion can cause disease. It also states that some emotions are symptoms of an illness.

We have found that Chinese medicine frequently helps people with emotional problems — even when the emotional issues are not the presenting complaint. Often a change results from treating the Organ associated with the person's underlying constitutional type. As the person's energy becomes stronger this in turn gives her or him a better emotional balance. This is an advantageous spiral — the *more* healthy we are, the easier it is to have 'normal' emotions which in turn helps us to be healthy.

Of course, the opposite also happens. The *less* healthy we are, the harder it is to balance our emotions which, in turn, can make us less well. This is a negative and downward spiral as opposed to a beneficial and upward one. For example, one patient said it was clear that the more stressed she was and the angrier she got, the worse her irritable bowel syndrome became. Of course, the cause and effect went both ways — the worse her irritable bowel syndrome, the more stressed, depressed and angry she became. When she came for treatment, she had rectal bleeding and was already on cortico-steroid drugs. The doctor said the next step would be surgery and the removal of some of her colon.

Fortunately for this woman, Chinese medicine treatments cleared her problems. She also felt more balanced emotionally. Having had Chinese medicine treatment she found that she was able effortlessly to deal with previously difficult situations. This is an example of the positive effect Chinese medicine often has on the emotions.

With other cases, we have found that treatment has helped patients to feel better in many ways but they then get stuck in recurring negative mental or emotional states. These can neutralize the previous positive effects of the treatment. If this is the case, we have found that it is helpful, *as well as* using Chinese medicine, to work with exercises appropriate to the person's type. A change of beliefs, values, attitudes and mental habits can release us from these recurring negative states and thus create better health. So when, as practitioners, we wanted to say 'Stop worrying and your energy will be more balanced', we found there are ways to put such a recommendation into practice.

This book is not just for you to read. You will also need to engage with it. After reading it, please ponder and make some guesses as to your constitutional type.

Then, you can embark on the set of exercises for your type. These exercises are not onerous or difficult and many are easy. For other exercises you may need to use your mind in new ways which may seem different or even awkward at first.

By reading about the different types and working through the relevant exercises we hope you will gain some useful insights into your internal world and thus create change in your life. Please note, however, that this book is not aimed at replacing treatment by a qualified practitioner of Chinese medicine or a trained therapist or counsellor — in fact we hope that by reading it you will feel like exploring Chinese medicine, or therapies such as NLP.

If you use these exercises, please do so with commitment, and do them gradually and repetitively. Results accumulate. We believe that you will definitely find the exercises much easier than simply stopping whatever emotions are helping to make you less well. We wish you the best of luck and would be happy to hear from you via our publisher.

NOTES

1   For many more examples of how our 'thinking' can change our experience, particularly examples of the effect of how we 'represent' something to ourselves, see Bandler, Richard; 1985; *Using Your Brain — For a Change*. The book is easy to read and often quite amusing. It is an edited transcript of a seminar and is almost jargon-free.

2   In the bibliography we have a special section on Qigong. The Chinese books, as opposed to the Western ones, use Qigong exercises as a form of treatment and they are incorporated into what is referred to in China as TCM, Traditional Chinese Medicine.

Chapter 1

THE FIVE ELEMENTS, CONSTITUTIONAL TYPES AND THE EMOTIONS

A long-term study at York University[1] has confirmed what many of us already intuitively know — that our negative emotions can cause disease. Psychologists tracked the progress of thousands of young students over a thirteen-year period.

At the beginning of the study, each student was monitored over the course of two terms. Tests gauged their personality, how they coped with stress and how healthy they were.

From the study the researchers found that emotions had an important effect on whether we get ill. The students who were emotionally balanced were *less* likely to become ill. On the other hand, the ones who:

+ dwelt on the past
+ were unable to take in support from others
+ got irritable from working too hard
+ found it difficult to express their feelings, or
+ were unable to remain cool in difficult situations

were *more* likely to become ill.

The illnesses varied from headaches to heart troubles, but it was found that the people who were most often in these negative states were likely to have more serious illnesses. The researchers noted something that Chinese medicine has known for over two thousand years. This is, that negative emotions place us under a kind of permanent stress which causes us to become unhealthy.

In this book we will be discussing this obvious truth, that repetitive negative emotional states cause us to become ill and conversely, that regular, positive and balanced emotions can help to keep us well.[2]

This chapter will introduce us to the Chinese view of health, disease and our emotions. It will also explain how these relate to Chinese Five Element theory and the Five Element types. This chapter will also give us a thorough background to all aspects of the Five Element types. This includes a brief history, their relationship to our Organs, how our constitutional type originates and an overview of the positive and negative capacities of the types. We will also look in greater depth at how we become ill and how we are affected by our emotions. Before we go any further, however, let's look at how the Chinese view disease.

CHINESE MEDICINE AND DISEASE

Chinese medicine teaches that there are three main areas which cause disease. These are called External, Internal and Miscellaneous causes.[3] The External causes relate to how the climate can make us ill. The Miscellaneous ones are mostly to do with how our lifestyle can affect us. It is the Internal ones, however, which we are dealing with in this book. This is because they are concerned with our emotions.

The Internal causes of disease were first noted in Chinese texts over two thousand years ago. They are clearly an even more important cause of disease in today's society than they were at that time.

You may be wondering what the emotions have got to do with the Five Elements and the Five Element 'types'.

THE FIVE ELEMENT 'TYPES'

The five main constitutional types are based around what is known as the theory of the Five Elements. Along with Yin and Yang, which are the two prime forces of the universe, Five Element theory underpins the whole of Chinese medicine.

Each of these Five Elements is associated with two main organs. We will discuss these organs and Elements in greater depth in this chapter and the later ones. All of us are born with one Element which is constitutionally slightly more imbalanced than the others.[4] This imbalance causes us to have repetitive negative states or difficulties expressing certain emotions.

If we have an imbalance in the Element known as 'Wood', for example, this is connected with the Liver and Gall Bladder organs. The associated emotions have to do with anger and assertion. An imbalance on the other hand in the Lungs and the 'Metal Element' will tend us more towards emotions connected with grief and loss.

By knowing and understanding our constitutional imbalance or 'type' we can know where our main emotional imbalance lies. *This is important because it enables us to specify the key areas where greater awareness and work on ourselves will pay the greatest dividends.* If, for example, the inability to grieve is a key factor, then 'working on our anger' is not as useful as responding to our diminished capacity for grief. After all, much of the anger may be coming from the inability to experience or express our grief.

In order to understand these types better we'll now find out more about the Five Elements.

WHAT ARE THE FIVE ELEMENTS?

As we said earlier, the Five Elements along with Yin and Yang are an important underlying structure of Chinese medicine. Five Element theory says that the energy of the world can be divided into five movements or processes which are sometimes also called phases or Elements. We will use the term 'Element' as it is the one most commonly used.

The Elements are: Fire, Earth, Metal, Water and Wood. They are the energetic substances or processes out of which the world is made. Each Element is defined as having a set of associations. For example, some of the associations are a Yin and a Yang Organ, a colour, a sound in the voice, a season, a taste, an odour, a direction and a climate. Through these associations arises a Five Element language to describe the world.

The Elements connect to each other via two cycles illustrated by the arrows. The cycles emphasize how aware the Chinese are of the interconnectedness of the Organs. Below is a diagram of the Five Elements and their generating and controlling cycles. Figure 1 shows the main associations of each Element.

THE FIRE ELEMENT
Heart; Small Intestine;
Pericardium; Triple Burner;
red; joy; scorched; summer;
south; heat; bitter

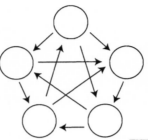

THE WOOD ELEMENT
Liver; Gall Bladder; green;
anger; shouting; rancid; spring;
east; wind; sour

THE EARTH ELEMENT
Spleen; Stomach; yellow;
sympathy/worry; singing;
fragrant; late summer; centre;
damp; sweet

THE WATER ELEMENT
Kidney; Bladder; blue/black;
fear; groaning; putrid; winter;
north; cold; salty

THE METAL ELEMENT
Lungs; Large Intestine; white;
grief; weeping; rotten; autumn;
west; dryness; pungent

Figure 1: THE FIVE ELEMENTS AND THEIR ASSOCIATIONS

HOW DO THE FIVE ELEMENT ASSOCIATIONS CONNECT?

Any situation in the world will always contain all of the Elements, but one will be dominant. As an example we'll assume it's a summer's day. The sun is bright and the temperature is scorching. People are gathered together and talking a lot, bright colours such as red appear in abundance and laughter resounds.

We would say from the description above, that of all the Elements, Fire is in the ascendant. Why? Because summer, heat, speech, laughter and the colour red are all associations of Fire. So is the heart. And so is the emotion joy.

The Five Element theory is a way of connecting many aspects of the world. We can use these to determine which Element is to the fore in a situation and which Elements are in the background.

HOW DID THE CHINESE USE THE FIVE ELEMENT THEORY?

The theory of the Five Elements was originated by a Chinese philosopher, Tsou Yen, a few hundred years before the birth of Christ. Tsou Yen is thought to be the founder of Chinese scientific thought. In his first writings, he described the movement from one Element to another. This was especially with regard to the change in power from one dynastic ruler to another. His political advice and insights became highly sought after. He was consulted by the various powerful lords, emperors and feudal rulers at a time when China was a group of warring states.

Over time, however, the Five Element theory was used in agriculture, war-making, and many other practical arts as well as political organization and medicine. Some of the uses may seem rather unusual to us today, but for the Chinese they were always practical and useful in everyday life.[5]

In medicine, the Five Elements were used in a similar manner to the Yin-Yang theory. This was to determine the underlying causes of acute and chronic illnesses. We believe, however, that one of the Five Elements' most successful uses lies in determining the patient's deepest Elemental imbalance or 'constitutional type'. This helps us to deal with chronic illness.

The way we, the authors, have been taught to determine constitutional type involves careful observation of the person's emotional state and an understanding of the emotion associated with each Element. Hence the connection in this book between the Element types and the emotions. So where did this system of finding an underlying imbalance originate?

A SHORT HISTORY OF THE FIVE ELEMENT TYPES

Five Element types were first mentioned in an ancient Chinese book called *The Yellow Emperor's Classic of Internal Medicine*.[6] People have changed since that time and the different types have been described in various ways throughout Chinese history.[7] Five Element types have also been described in other oriental countries such as Japan and Korea.[8]

The types which we describe in this book were taught to us by an acupuncture teacher called JR Worsley over twenty years ago.[9]

FINDING OUR FIVE ELEMENT TYPE

There are different ways of establishing which of the Elements is the one which is primarily imbalanced. The system we use, and describe in this book, starts with the notion of one Element being the weak link in the chain of the Five Elements. Because all of the Elements are linked, the Element which was originally imbalanced will affect all of the others. It will, however, also create certain recognizable characteristics in a person. These are described in the individual chapters on each type.

FINDING THE UNDERLYING CAUSE

Chinese medicine is an energetic medicine which means, among other things, that rather than just examining a person's body, we look for the underlying or energetic cause of a patient's problem.

We usually think that our everyday life is made up of a multitude of things, including events, thoughts, objects and people. On the other hand we can simplify a day's events by considering our basic needs and asking ourselves if they were satisfied. We can forget all the details of what happened today and say, 'Was today a good day?' This is another way of saying 'What's underneath all my concerns? What's important?'

The Chinese frequently look 'underneath it all' and ask what is happening to a person on a deeper level. For example, in Chinese medicine it is typical not only to address a patient's symptoms, but also to look for the energetic cause which underlies the symptoms. This is often referred to as the deeper cause.

Chinese medicine teaches that our 'Qi' (pronounced 'chee') underlies all of our functioning. It is the force which warms, moves, transforms and protects everything in our bodies and minds. The Five Elements describe five important phases or variations in this underlying Qi.

THE ORGANS AND THE FIVE ELEMENTS

We mentioned earlier that each of the Five Elements has two Organs associated with it (apart from the Fire Element which has four). We'll now take a deeper look at them. One of the Organs is a 'Yin' Organ and the other is a 'Yang' Organ and they are 'paired' together.

The quality of Yang is more active and external than Yin which is more still and internal. Consequently the Yin Organs lie deeper inside the body and are concerned more with storing or retaining. The Yang Organs have more to do with transformation, movement and elimination. Below is a list of the Yin and Yang Organs associated with each Element.

Element	Yin Organ	Yang Organ
Wood	Liver	Gall Bladder
Fire	Heart	Small Intestine
	Pericardium	Triple Burner
Earth	Spleen	Stomach
Metal	Lungs	Large Intestine
Water	Kidney	Bladder

We often refer to these Organs as an 'Organ system'. By this we mean the Yin and Yang Organ as well as a number of other functions connected with each Organ. Because we are talking about the Chinese rather than the Western understanding of an Organ, which is similar but also very different in emphasis, we will also capitalize the name of an Organ or Organ system when we are referring to the Chinese understanding. These are discussed in greater detail in the individual chapters on each type.

HOW DID OUR ELEMENTAL IMBALANCE ORIGINATE?

It is believed that the Organs of one of the Elements is slightly imbalanced from the time we are born. We therefore call it our constitutional imbalance or type. The Organ system affects the healthy functioning of both our bodies *and* our minds. Where the Organs are constitutionally weaker, this will have an important effect on our personality as well as our physical health. A child born with weak Lungs will have a different life from one born with strong Lungs but weak Kidneys.

Because in this book, we are giving the greatest emphasis to the effect of the constitutional weakness on the 'emotions', it is important to say how the word 'emotions' is being used. We are using the word in its widest sense. It is more the predisposition to feel a certain way and take up certain attitudes to the world around us. We will talk more about what an emotion is in a few moments.

OUR ELEMENTAL IMBALANCE AND OUR EMOTIONS IN OUR EARLY LIFE

We have now described how one of our Organ systems is weaker from birth. The weakest one will create a tendency towards a different set of emotions experienced early in life. If it is the Heart, for instance, then the emotions we experience will be around joy and sadness. The Organs and the emotions associated with each Element are:

Element	Emotion
Fire	Joy/Sadness
Earth	Sympathy/Worry
Metal	Grief/Loss
Water	Fear
Wood	Anger

These different emotional imbalances lead to the development of different personalities, built around our different values and expectations of the world. We can put this into a diagram:

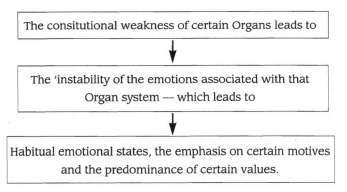

The consitutional weakness of certain Organs leads to

↓

The 'instability of the emotions associated with that Organ system — which leads to

↓

Habitual emotional states, the emphasis on certain motives and the predominance of certain values.

THE ORGANS AND THE EMOTIONS

Saying that an Organ system is 'connected to' or 'makes an emotion possible' may sound odd. It is not a belief we have in the West. In the West, for example, the lungs are not thought to connect with our emotions. The Five Element associations, however, say that the Lungs and grief are connected. Well-balanced Lungs can lead to the healthy expression of grief.

From our clinical experience we have seen that patients with weak Lungs often have difficulty with the expression of healthy and normal grief. When a patient's Lungs are strengthened by treatment or exercises, their ability 'to experience grief' improves. The effect of the Lungs on the expression of grief is particularly important when the weakness of the Organ is constitutional. Hence the significance of the types.

What we mean exactly by 'grief' and the ability 'to experience grief' will be clearer in the chapter on the Metal type. For the moment, the notion of an emotion overlaps with many other parts of our personality. In the chapters on each Element we describe how at the core of a person there are five key 'major concerns'. Although all of us have a wide range of other motivating factors in our lives, we all have some which are more important than others.

Why is this so important? It is important because it specifies which are our core weaknesses, our core strengths and, most definitely, our core sensitivities. Knowing these suggests the most fruitful place to work on ourselves.

CORE MOTIVATORS — EACH PERSON HAS A *BIG* ONE

So how do we describe these 'big' motivating factors in our lives. We need to go back now and take a couple of simple steps. The first is from the Elements to their associations.

For example, the associations of the Fire Element are:

- the Heart as an Organ
- joy as an emotion
- red as a colour (as it appears on the face)
- scorched as an odour (not 'body odour', but it comes from the body)
- laughing as a sound in the voice (not literally a laugh)
- and many other aspects including a taste, a season and a climate.

Of these associations, the most important for us are the Organs, the emotions and the capacity for emotional expression which a healthy Organ gives us. These positive functions or capacities arise when the Organs are working well.

WHAT ARE THE POSITIVE EMOTIONAL CAPACITIES OF EACH ELEMENT?

Below is a simple table which describes these capacities. Because we are keeping them simple they are described very generally. Of course they vary enormously in the way they manifest.

Element	Main Organ	The Emotional Capacity this Element Gives us
Fire	Heart	The capacity to feel joy; the ability to give and receive warmth and love with varying degrees of emotional closeness.

Earth	Stomach and Spleen	The capacity to take in support and nourishment as well as to support and nourish others appropriately.
Metal	Lung	The capacity to feel loss and to move on; the ability to take in quality and richness in order to feel complete.
Water	Kidney	The capacity to feel fear and to sense and assess risk and respond appropriately.
Wood	Liver	The capacity to be appropriately assertive; to have structures and boundaries which enable us to grow and develop.

These are the capacities of the Element when it is working well. Another important way of looking at these capacities is to see them from their negative side. We might wonder, for example, what kind of experiences we might have if one Element is not working well?

WHAT EMOTIONAL EXPERIENCES DOES A CONSTITUTIONALLY WEAK ELEMENT LEAD TO?

When an Element is imbalanced, the capacities associated with it are diminished. A diminished capacity leads to certain sorts of experience. The descriptions below describe the kinds of things we might say if the Organ is imbalanced.

The descriptions are very general and could apply to us at any stage in our life. This could be anything from a pre-verbal infant to an adult who may well be reacting with mixed emotions rather than a simple state of mind. In the individual chapters, we will be giving more details and examples of these.

Element	*Main Organ*	*Typical Negative Experiences When This Element is Weak*
Fire	Heart	Hurt, abandonment, feeling unloved, people are not loving and warm, 'Am I not lovable?'
Earth	Stomach and Spleen	Not going to be fed, others getting fed before me, not protected or held or supported, 'No-one to look after me'.
Metal	Lung	Not recognized, acknowledged, 'No-one knows I am here', 'Why do I feel that something is missing?'

Water	Kidney	Frightened and not reassured, 'No-one tells me realistically that I'll be safe', 'Can I trust?'
Wood	Liver	'I feel angry, frustrated and violated', 'I'm no longer clear about what I want', 'I don't know what's right'.

The negative experiences which are associated with a weakness in one of our Elements will affect the development of our personality. A Fire type, for example, will have weak Heart energy and be more likely to have many early experiences which come under the general heading of 'not feeling loved' and 'feeling unlovable'. It is easy then to develop a personality with habitual emotional states which reflect these experiences. These experiences frequently turn into beliefs, for instance, that 'I am unlovable'. This in turn begins to create our experience of the world. For example, if I believe I am unlovable, then I do not truly accept the love of others as, after all, 'I *am* unlovable'.

Experiences of not being loved can then lead a Fire type to develop various ways of coping. These could include:

♦ Closing down to close relationships and moving more towards superficial, social or 'party' type relationships.

♦ Being determined to maintain a close relationship at any cost with an over-valuing of any hint of warmth and affection.

♦ Closing down to any close relationship but focusing on some other method of gaining warmth, e.g. being famous, successful, making others laugh.

♦ Entering close relationships, being hurt or at least anticipating hurt, pulling away to safety, only to repeat the same pattern many times over.

Behind these behaviours is a reaction to the negative experiences which arose from the initial constitutional weakness. 'I felt unloved, so in the future I will protect myself by ...'. In each of the chapters on the types, we will look at these basic capacities and the negative experiences which can easily arise and in adulthood cause us emotional problems.

WHAT HAS BEING HEALTHY GOT TO DO WITH OUR CONSTITUTIONAL IMBALANCE?

All types can be healthy or unhealthy.

So why does one person end up more healthy and the other more unhealthy? We assume that the common sense reasons are probably the true ones. Firstly, some people are born healthier than others. In addition, children who have their basic emotional needs satisfied will tend to be healthier. People who have sought insight into themselves and made choices based on these insights are also more likely to be healthy.

It is clear that as well as constitutional type, upbringing and personal awareness are the keys to emotional good or bad health. As we cannot go back and change our history, we need to change our awareness, make better decisions and change our beliefs about our history. That is where the exercises come in. The purpose of the exercises is to increase awareness and ultimately to help us to make better choices.

IS A TYPE ALWAYS BASED IN WEAKNESS?

Concentrating on the negative experiences which evolve from our constitutional imbalance suggests that it is just the label for an illness. This is not so. Most people have both the negative and positive aspects of their type in their personality.

Although each of the types *does* have a limited set of concerns it is also true that they will develop special sensitivities and special abilities. For example, the Fire type will have experiences around being unloved. Love and warmth become important. This can lead to a highly developed sensitivity to people and a capacity to understand and meet other's needs as well as their own. When we discuss each type in detail we will refer to how, typically, a type will have certain good qualities or 'virtues'.

Negative experiences do play a role in the formation of anyone's personality, but having a 'constitutional type' is not the label for a sickness.

WHAT IS AN EMOTION?

We have now come full circle through the Five Elements and our Constitutional type and back to the emotions. We have spoken about emotions as if everyone understands what we mean. Psychologists do not necessarily agree about what an emotion is. Experience has taught us to think of an emotion not as an isolated thing, but as having many parts to it.

An Emotion is Made up of Many Different Parts

1 *Sensations:* 'a rush of energy moving up in my chest', 'a tightening in my stomach', 'a sinking in the chest, right down to my navel'.
2 *Thoughts or spoken words:* 'I feel so good about you', 'I hate it when he does that', 'I am so disappointed'.
3 *Expression:* facial expression, gestures, body posture, voice tone.
4 *Behaviour:* reaching out to touch someone. Clenching fists, slumping and letting the head drop.
5 *The situation and roles:* we have to take into consideration whether we are on stage, in a classroom, with a close friend or talking to a shop assistant.

Because an emotion is made up of parts, it can occur in different ways and to varying degrees. The emotion associated with Wood is anger, but this really begins as a normal assertion of ourselves and then, when we are blocked, we can experience frustration, upset, irritation, anger, rage and finally we go, as people say, 'ballistic'. As the emotion escalates, the parts combine in different ways. All these can be associated with the Wood Element. We do not, of course, have to be a Wood type to get angry.

HOW DO WE KNOW SOMEONE IS ANGRY?

The way we recognize that someone is angry is by their use of words, their expression, behaviour and the context in which they are reacting. We don't know, however, what their thoughts or sensations are. For this reason, we can easily disagree about what someone is feeling. We can even disagree with the person who is having the feelings. For example, we can imagine the following conversation:

'I am *not* angry. How can you be so stupid?'

'Well, you are shouting, clenching your fists and saying you are going to wring his neck. And you *look* angry.'

'You shut up.' (Shouting) 'I am not bloody angry. I am hurt!'

WHAT IS THE DIFFERENCE BETWEEN FEELING ANGRY AND BEING AN ANGRY PERSON?

In everyday life we may look at someone and think 'they are angry'. We would recognize this by using some of the 'parts' described above — especially, their words, expression and behaviour. Saying someone is an angry person is simply saying that they get angry a lot and maybe on occasions when others, in the same situation, wouldn't. In this book, we are usually talking about a person's tendency to have the same emotions, over and over again — like the angry person.

HOW DO EMOTIONS CAUSE DISEASE?

At the beginning of this chapter we said that the emotions are called an Internal cause of disease. Western research is supporting the ancient Chinese view that disruptive emotions negatively affect our health. So how does this happen?

In the first place, emotions are natural and not all emotions are causes of disease. Part of the understanding of the Five Elements is that we need to be nourished emotionally and we need to express feelings. All of the Elements have qualities which nourish them and fulfil their basic needs.

Element	Basic Need
Fire	Love, warmth, joy.
Earth	Support, nourishment, care.
Metal	Recognition, acknowledgement of self.
Water	Safety, reassurance, stability.
Wood	Boundaries and structure to facilitate growth.

Being nourished will involve feelings. We feel warm when we are loved, secure when supported, satisfied when acknowledged, relaxed when safe and excited when our boundaries and vision are clear. Whatever the feelings, it is natural for us to have them when our Elemental needs are satisfied.

It is also natural on occasion to have negative feelings. If we are abruptly and inexplicably abandoned by a partner, it would be natural to feel unloved and devastated. The same applies to many situations. So if this is natural, when do emotions cause illness?

In adult life, a feeling which is too strong can cause illness. Being involved in a disaster where our lives are threatened and those close to us die, can produce such overwhelming feelings that leaves us unable to resume a normal flow of energy.

Something like this, although not externally devastating, can happen when we are young and not be noticed by those around us. For example, our mother is ill and consequently absent shortly after birth; at an impressionable age we have a teacher with inappropriately high expectations; we are the first born and a sibling arrives unexpectedly. Any of these events can seem catastrophic from the point of view of a child. The result can be that some emotions we feel day by day can make us ill. These emotions have several characteristics:

- ♦ They are repetitive or prolonged, occurring over and over again and seem to be a part of our personality.
- ♦ They are generated from inside us, via memories, although an external event might trigger them.
- ♦ They are often experienced as unpleasant.
- ♦ We often feel passive when undergoing these emotions, as if they happen *to us* and we cannot do anything about them.

An overwhelming one-off emotion may make us ill. Consistently, however, the emotions causing disease are the everyday, repetitive, negative feelings over which we feel we have no control. These arise from our own internal way of experiencing the world.

SO, AGAIN, WHAT IS AN EMOTION?

We said before that an emotion is made up of many parts. The Chinese would also describe an emotion as simply the flow of Qi or energy. Ideally, this flow should always be free and never blocked. It is natural for emotions to arise, flow smoothly, reach a peak and dissipate. However, the emotions described above — which are repetitive, generated mainly from the inside, unpleasant and seemingly outside our control — are based on blockage. When the Qi is blocked, stagnation occurs. A pond which is no longer fed by flowing streams begins to stagnate. Stuck emotions cause the Qi of the body to stagnate and illness results.

For example, grief which is held in the chest means that the natural flow of energy in the chest is inhibited. Fear which is held in the lower back stops the flow of blood to the kidneys. Anger which tightens the chest area can reduce blood flow to the heart. Even love or joy which we hold back makes the pond stagnant.

THE REST OF THE BOOK

The next ten chapters consist of a chapter for each constitutional type followed by a chapter giving the exercises for that type. There are five different types: Wood, Fire, Earth, Metal and Water types. Each chapter on a type is designed both to describe the type and to give us the background in Chinese medicine to help us to understand the type. The purpose of the exercise chapters is to give us ways to grow and develop and achieve more balanced emotions. The rest of this chapter offers you some guidance to reading the book.

HOW TO DISCOVER YOUR TYPE

You can go about discovering your type in one of two ways. First, you may decide to read the whole book or chapters 2, 4, 6, 8 and 10 which describe the five main types. You may then notice which of the types describes you the best. Alternatively, you may wish to fill in the questionnaire at the end of the book and find out which type gains the highest score. You can then read the associated chapter and see if it 'fits'. Of course you may also wish to do both!

If you decide to take the first route suggested, this is a useful way to gain insights into your type. As you read chapters 2, 4, 6, 8 and 10, you may decide that the characteristics of one of the types describe you well. If this is the case it is strongly possible that this is your constitutional type. You may gain greater understanding of yourself by reading the chapter and also from carrying out the exercises associated with your type. Doing these exercises will help you quickly to pinpoint and work on a number of your key issues. Thus you can uncover and deal with many important areas for your growth and development. It will also enable you to consider the ways in which those around you are different or similar in the way they think, feel and go about their daily lives. This awareness of others can be an important benefit of knowing about the different types.

The second route to discovering your type is the questionnaire. You will find this in Chapter 12 on page 218. The questions are asked from many different perspectives in order for you to gain a clear idea of your Elemental type. *Please remember though that no questionnaire is foolproof.* If the results of the questionnaire indicate that you are a certain type and the associated chapter is a good description of you, then you have probably found your type. If, on the other hand, it does not describe you well, then you can assume that the questionnaire has not given you an accurate result. In this case you may wish to read the descriptions of the other types too. If you then feel more in tune with another type then please read both types again carefully and assess for yourself which one describes you the best.

Some of you may already know your type because you have visited an acupuncturist who has told you that one of the Elements is the key focus of your treatment. Your acupuncturist may even suggest that you read this book in order to gain greater insight into the Element or suggest that you do some of these exercises.

I Relate to Many of the Elements as I Read This Book. What Should I Do?

When you read about the types you may find that more than one of them describe some aspects of your character. This is natural as we are a combination of all five types. Because we have our own unique balance of all of the Elements there are times when many of the main characteristics described in the chapters may sound vaguely familiar. However, when you come to the chapter which describes your constitutional type you may realise that this particular type stands out from the others. It will usually provide a much more accurate description of you and you may even have a gut feeling which says, 'Yes, this is my type. It fits me.' The fit can be especially accurate in terms of the emotion associated with your type and some of the big issues and the responses to them.

Help, I Can't Decide Between Two Types

As we said earlier we have all of the Five elements within us so you may resonate strongly with more than one type. Some of you may find that two or more Elements describe you strongly. If this is the case both Elements are probably important even though only one of them is your constitutional type. You may find that you benefit from doing the exercises associated with both types. Alternatively, you may find you benefit from doing the exercises for one type more than the other. In this case it might indicate that this Element is your constitutional type.

I Think I Know my Type But I'd Also Like to do Some of the Exercises for the Other Types

We have done our best to identify exercises which will particularly benefit each of the types. Many of the exercises are, in some contexts, however, useful for other types. For example, 'Focusing' from the Wood exercises on page 43 is useful for many different types and the exercises on forming relationships which are in the chapter on the Fire exercises (page 84) are useful for many of us at certain times of our lives and when we want to improve our relationships. The exercise 'Dealing with Loss' on page 172 is included with the grief exercises. This exercise is useful for anyone who has suffered a loss of any kind. Please feel free to do exercises not associated with your type if you recognize that they might benefit you.

The purpose of the exercise chapters is to give us ways to grow and develop and achieve more balanced emotions. Once you know your type we would suggest you read through the exercises associated with that chapter first and then plan your approach to working through them.   •

Good luck. We hope you enjoy the book and benefit from the exercises!

Notes

1 Unpublished paper, D Roger, Y Birks, A Forbes, B Najarian: *Toxic and Non-toxic Personalities — Individual Differences in Susceptibility to Illness*; University of York, 1998. This paper was presented at the 9th European Conference on Personality at the University of Surrey in July 1998.

2 If you have any doubts about repetitive negative emotions causing illness, then you can consult the growing base of Western research which supports the ancient Chinese view. Some of this is easily available in Goleman, Daniel, 1995: *Emotional Intelligence*; Bloomsbury Publishing, London. This book was on the bestseller list in 1997. In chapter 11, Goleman gives many examples of the research done in the West on the connection between emotional disturbance and illness.

3 See Hicks, Angela: *The Five Laws for Healthy Living*; Thorsons, 1998, for a practical discussion of the Chinese wisdom on how to develop a healthy lifestyle. The book in your hands concentrates on the internal causes of disease whilst *The Five Laws for Healthy Living* also gives an account of external and miscellaneous (lifestyle) causes of disease.

4 We know that everyone has an imbalance in one of the Five Elements from early on in their lives. Discussion continues as to the nature/nurture issue, that is, how much we are born with and how much arises during our early childhood. The authors believe we are born with the imbalance.

5 You can read more about the ancient Chinese use of Five Element theory in Needham, Joseph: *The Shorter Science and Civilisation in China 1*, pages 142—57.

6 This book first appeared around 200 BC. It appears to be written by more than one author and it has been available as a source of inspiration continuously since publication. It does give solutions to medical problems, but it is much more a discussion of the fundamental questions of medicine. There are many different translations and it has different titles in English, e.g. *The Yellow Emperor's Classic of Medicine*. See bibliography for these.

7 See for example, Koo, Linda Chih-ling, 1982: *Nourishment of Life*; pp 127–31.

8 See Eckman, Peter, 1996: *In the Footsteps of the Yellow Emperor*; pp 208–9.

9 JR Worsley called the primary imbalance of a person the 'Causative Factor'. This is the name which is most often used by practitioners who use this Five Element style of acupuncture treatment and it suggests that the constitutional weakness of the organs has an important effect on both our health and our emotional expression.

Chapter 2

THE WOOD TYPE - ASSERTING OURSELVES

DELIA IS A WOOD TYPE

At work everyone admires Delia. She's dynamic and efficient and if we want someone to take responsibility we know we can rely on her. 'I've always been the kind of person who likes to get things done', she told us, 'In fact with other people I have to sometimes hold myself back because it's so easy for me to jump in and organize them. I tend to find myself in leadership roles, I suppose it's because I put myself forward. I can often see things that others don't notice. In fact if someone says something isn't possible I'll rise to the challenge and do battle. Sometimes it's just bloody mindedness to show that it can be done.'

In her social life Delia is just as dynamic. She belongs to many organizations which she hopes will help to change the world and make it a better place to live. One organization is Amnesty International: 'I get outraged when I hear people are being treated unjustly. It really makes my blood boil.'

Delia's facial colour has a greenish tinge to it and she speaks with a precise and clipped voice. These, along with her assertive disposition are indications that she is a Wood type. Acupuncture treatment helped her to deal with occasional tightness in the chest and migraines and abdominal pain prior to her period — she says she feels 'smoother' and 'better in herself' generally. She also worked on herself using some of the exercises in this book. One particularly useful exercise was learning to experience a situation from another's point of view.

In this chapter we will be looking at the characteristics of a Wood type. As you read, you may appreciate why Delia is a Wood type and understand more about her underlying motivations. We will start by looking at the Wood Element in Chinese medicine.

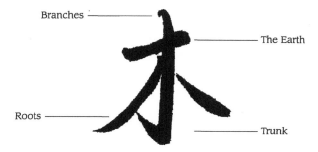

Branches

The Earth

Roots

Trunk

Figure 2: THE CHINESE CHARACTER FOR WOOD

THE WOOD ELEMENT IN NATURE

The Chinese character for Wood is Mu (see character drawn above). This character represents a tree. The vertical line is the trunk and root of the tree; the horizontal line is the earth. The line at the top represents branches. The lower lines are the roots which clearly form the main part of the picture.[1]

The Wood Element is associated with Spring and the time when all vegetation begins to grow. We can imagine an oak tree and its beginning as an acorn. The acorn begins to grow under the ground and pushes outwards and upwards. Already, at the start, the acorn knows where it is going. It is destined to become an oak tree. Acorns do not become maples, birches or scotch pines. The blueprint or plan of an oak tree is already contained in the acorn.

When growth begins, an impediment, like a stone lying on the earth above the acorn, will be pushed out of the way as the tree first emerges. Pushing the stone out of the way is not an aggressive act. It is just that 'an acorn does what an acorn has to do'. The acorn emerges and over time, given suitable conditions, grows into a tall, green-leaved oak.

As we discuss this Element, we will see several connections between how an acorn transforms into an oak and how the Wood Element enables us to develop into mature human beings.

THE BACKGROUND TO WOOD IN CHINESE MEDICINE

Introduction

The Wood Element consists of the notion of Wood itself — as expressed in the character and the acorn — and all the Wood associations. The key associations are:

Organs   Liver and Gall Bladder
Spirit   Hun – the mental-spiritual aspect of the Wood Element
Colour   Green
Sound   Shouting
Emotion   Anger
Odour   Rancid

These associations are discussed in more detail in this section. Familiarity with them will enable us to recognize Wood types and understand the connections between the Organ functions and mental processes described later.

The Organs of the Wood Element

The Chinese described the functions of the Organs differently from the way they are described in the West. In the West, we have a physical and functional description. The Chinese gave both a metaphorical description and also a functional description in terms of 'Qi' (the energy of the body and mind) and Blood.[2] They also attributed various mental and spiritual functions to the Organs, for example, for Wood, the spirit is called the 'Hun'.

The Liver and Gall Bladder and its Mental-Spiritual Aspect

Metaphorically the Liver is said to be the 'General' who makes plans and the Gall Bladder is the 'Decision maker'.[3] This means that our ability to organize, plan and make decisions is related to the well-being of the Liver and Gall Bladder. The Liver and Gall Bladder's capacity to organize, plan and make decisions is in the service of the 'Hun' or 'Ethereal' Soul. This is the mental-spiritual aspect of the Liver. Our Hun is responsible for our 'life plan', sense of purpose and sense of direction.

Ordinarily this process will be smooth and completely unconscious. In times of difficulty, however, the planning process can come to the surface. Jacqueline, a Wood type, told us:

I'm aware that if I don't have a specific forward direction, it's easy for me to get depressed. Once I have a direction again I'm happy. I think I'm over-directed sometimes and I *have* to have something I can see ahead. Seeing ahead of me is so important that I tend to be two jumps ahead of myself and take on too much.

Our Smoothly Flowing Qi

As well as being the 'General', the Liver is said to *make the Qi of the body and mind flow smoothly*. To help us to understand this function more clearly we can think of a baby sitting on the floor. The baby notices a soft toy and reaches out, picks it up, shakes it up and down, gurgles and laughs and then lets go. From noticing the toy to dropping it is a smooth process.

Suppose, however, that just as the baby reaches out for the toy someone shouts 'No'. The baby might tense up, pull back and look towards the 'No'. The energy is interrupted and flows jerkily. After the first 'No', the baby might again see the toy, but hesitate and look around. The smooth and natural flow of Qi has been broken.

At first the baby's smooth flow is interrupted from the outside. With sufficient interruptions, however, the Liver will no longer be able to smooth the Qi from the inside. Later in life this can produce a wide variety of symptoms — from moodiness and depression to irregular periods, period pains and clots in the menstrual blood. These are expanded in the section on the symptoms of the Liver and Gall Bladder.

Storing the Blood

A second function of the Liver is 'to store the Blood'. 'Blood' in Chinese medicine is similar to that in Western medicine. It moistens and nourishes all parts of the body. When we are resting, Chinese medicine teaches that the Blood goes to the Liver and replenishes it. When, on the other hand, we are active it travels to our extremities so that we can move.

When the Liver is not storing the Blood adequately, we will not be nourished in our extremities or on the outside of the body. Symptoms which arise can include numb limbs, pins and needles or breaking nails. Weak or blurred vision can also occur as the Blood is not nourishing the eyes.

THESE SYMPTOMS MAY ARISE WHEN THE LIVER AND GALL BLADDER ARE WEAK OR OBSTRUCTED

Some of these symptoms are more physical and some more mental or of the spirit. Chinese medicine being 'energetic' did not make this an important distinction.

Difficulties with planning, making decisions and 'having a future'. Nervousness, timidity and a lack of courage and initiative. Eye problems, e.g. blurred vision, 'floaters', specific eye diseases and headaches with mild to severe pain. Muscle tension, held-in feelings, repressed anger, emotional outbursts, depression, moodiness, feeling emotionally overwhelmed and over-sensitive and having difficulty in making plans. Upset digestion with belching and regurgitation, allergies, nausea, vomiting or an inability to digest fats. Tightness in the chest which may also manifest as a breathing difficulty and discomfort under the ribs. Tiredness, dry skin, muscular weakness and spasms, mild dizziness, pins and needles and dry and brittle nails and poor sleep. Period-related problems such as pre-menstrual tension and pain.

Observable Signs of a Wood Type

Practitioners of Chinese medicine rely heavily on observable signs. Some key things that can be noticed about Wood types are:

♦ A light or bottle green colour at the side or under the eyes and around the mouth.
♦ A rancid odour similar to the smell of rancid butter.
♦ A 'clipped' sound within the voice where emphasis is placed on individual syllables, as if we spoke with barely held in anger.
♦ The person's emotional expression which we will deal with in a later section.

Posture, Gestures and Facial Expression

The face of a Wood type will often, although not necessarily, show indications of chronic anger or assertiveness. These may be two vertical lines between the eyebrows, tension of the lower eyelid and a tense jaw.

The eyes are the sense organ associated with Wood. Sometimes the eyes of a Wood type can have a hesitant quality, not quite looking at you and coming and going. Often, however, the Wood type's eyes are quite intense. They may almost be fierce, indicating some held-in anger, but they may just be very direct in the way they look.

Some Wood types have a body characteristic of compression or having been squeezed. This has probably resulted from holding in anger. If we imagine squeezing ourselves inwards or holding ourselves back it will make our body appear to be 'packed in' or compressed. Wood types may also look tense and have a tight musculature. Hilary told us:

> When I get frustrated I often feel tense under my ribs and also in my neck and shoulders. At those times I would love a good strong massage to loosen up.

Many Wood types use gestures such as pointing their index fingers, jerky movements or using closed fists. Some less assertive Wood types, however, will have very few gestures.

These observations help us to assess whether someone is a Wood type.

THE EMOTIONAL CAPACITY OF THE WOOD ELEMENT

The Wood Element gives us an overall capacity which strongly affects our emotional life. We can describe this in the following way.

- ♦ The capacity to be appropriately assertive.
- ♦ To have structures and boundaries which enable us to grow and develop.

Rules, Structures and Boundaries

Why are rules, structures and boundaries important? They allow us to manifest our 'Hun' or overall purpose. They give us a sense of order in our lives. They allow us to unfold our day-to-day and longer-term plans. Without appropriate rules, structure and boundaries our life is not workable.

When a child is born, there are few understood boundaries. If we have watched a young baby who notices its hand in front of its face without knowing whose hand it is, then we can understand that it takes time to develop boundaries.

At a very early age we discover different parts of our body. Later on we find out that our skin is the boundary between the inside and outside world. We also discover that our mothers or primary carers are different from us — we cannot control them in the way we seem to control ourselves.

Later we discover other differences — between *others'* toys and *my* toys, *work* time and *play* time, *bed* room and *living* room, *intimate* relationships and *professional* ones — and thus we discover various social boundaries. The boundaries produce structure and regulate our lives.

Flexible Boundaries and Assertiveness

In general, a good boundary is not air-tight and rigid. Like skin, a boundary should create separation and also allow some movement across it. Boundaries allow us to be both separate individuals as well being part of a partnership or group.

It is not necessary that everyone has the same set of boundaries. Boundaries range widely from that of our skin to, for example, the rules and procedures which govern a country. However, no human grows and develops without boundaries at all.

The capacity created by Wood is sometimes to accept existing rules and boundaries and sometimes to re-negotiate or develop new ones. This allows us to be appropriately assertive and to express ourselves in the external world.

If we have constitutionally imbalanced Wood we may be predisposed to more than our usual share of difficulties to do with rules, structures and boundaries. A healthy Wood Element will allow us to develop rules, structures and boundaries which encourage our growth and development.

EMOTIONS WE EXPERIENCE WHEN THE ABILITY IS IMPAIRED

When the acorn encountered the stone, it simply pushed it out of the way. When we are attempting to get somewhere and we are blocked, we often have an emotional response. We feel frustrated, possibly even angry and then we attempt to deal with the block.

But supposing our Wood Element is weak and our capacity to assert ourselves is less strong than it might be. What happens then? We end up more and more frequently feeling frustrated and unable to push things through to a resolution. Effectively, we experience more:

♦ Frustration and anger
♦ Ambivalence and indecision

We'll talk about each of these in turn.

Frustration and Anger

Frustration is a normal response to being blocked. When our Wood Element is healthy, this frustration leads to adaption, renewed effort, negotiation or creativity. When our Wood Element is weaker, the frustration easily escalates into ineffective anger and difficulty in adapting to existing rules, boundaries and structures — or finding new ones.

Although the emotion associated with Wood is usually labelled 'anger', the frustration of natural assertion has many degrees and a rich descriptive vocabulary. We might use words like: frustration, irritation, annoyance, gall, pique, resentment, fury, outrage, indignation, exasperation, rage or wrath to describe the degrees of how we feel. We might use various colloquialisms often implying the addition of heat and weaponry, e.g. 'blood boiling', 'blew my top', 'went ballistic'. All these states are a development from basic frustration and there are a great variety of ways to express them.

Here Hilary describes her extremes of anger:

I seem to have fluctuating moods. I can be easily angered or irritated or spontaneously happy as well. My mood changes a lot. When I get angry I feel intensely scrunched up inside and I can feel my mouth crumple up into a ball. Sometimes I feel I want to kill someone or I feel like throwing or smashing something. When it's gone it's a contrast and it's gone completely.

Simon describes a common experience for Wood types; wanting to express, but pulling back from showing the real feelings.

The other day on a bus, the driver was driving like a kamikaze pilot. I wanted to go and say 'you are driving *people* you know' and I kept holding back but wanting to say something. Once I start having a go about something I know I'll be doing it all the time, so I don't say anything.

SOME RESEARCH ABOUT ANGER

Research shows that getting angry can seriously damage our health. One study found that when people remembered and recounted an incident which made them angry, the pumping efficiency of their hearts dropped *on average by 5 per cent*. A 7 per cent drop is thought to be potentially dangerous![4]

Ambivalence and Indecision

The full venting of anger is only occasionally effective in getting us what we want and, even when it works, there may be negative side effects. So ambivalence and indecision are a natural progression from wanting to be angry, but at the same time not wanting to. Ambivalence or indecisiveness may feel awkward, but they will at least maintain personal and social contacts. The feelings of anger, of course, remain unexpressed and get stored somewhere in the body.

Wood types like Julia and Jacqueline find it hard to show their anger and frustration. Julia says:

I don't get angry when I should do, then I get angry with the wrong person. I might also cry if I feel angry. Eighty per cent of the time I might be experiencing anger but cry as well. I might not say anything when I'm angry but then it sits inside me and I think about it a lot and it festers.

Jacqueline told us:

I talk about my anger towards people but then I don't show it with the people I'm angry with and I back down. I appear to be assertive, but it takes a huge amount to manifest anger to their face.

Eleanor tells us about the difficulties she has making a decision:

I can think I've made a decision but because other options are there, I can't leave it alone. I can't rest with it properly. Other things keep popping up and I want to take everything into account. I see other people making clear decisions and not worrying about the 'ifs' and 'buts' anymore. For me other possibilities stay in the picture and it makes life difficult.

Ambivalence and indecision make it difficult to move forward in our day-to-day lives. If we return to the baby's natural reaching out for something, and appreciate that this normal urge can get transformed into indecision, how then can we recognize a distorted expression in everyday life?

EXCESSIVE ANGER AND OUR HEALTH

Research carried out by Dr Redford Williams at Duke University found that excessive anger was a higher predictor of dying young than smoking, high blood pressure and high cholesterol! He asked students at the medical school to fill in questionnaires and found those who scored highest on the test for hostility and anger were seven times more likely to have died by the time they were fifty than those with lower scores.[5]

Recognizing the Emotion of a Wood Type in Everyday Life

The Wood types will often manifest anger which is not appropriate to a situation or fail to be angry when it is appropriate. This means having a keen sense of 'social rules' as these often dictate what is appropriate or inappropriate. For example, the following are a violation of unwritten rules:

♦ Forgetting to phone to cancel an important meeting.
♦ Disclosing information which is personal and is understood by both parties to be confidential.
♦ Buying a second hand car, then bouncing the cheque.

In each of these cases, a boundary has been broken and requires some sort of response.

Wood types, however, may not be able to respond with normal assertiveness. They might, for example, fail to react when a boundary has been violated or, alternatively, will be responding with anger and assertion even when they have not been unjustifiably violated.

In the first case, we will notice a person describing an event and in the back of our minds we will be thinking, 'I'd be angry about that!' In the second, we may be puzzled as to why the person is so angry and noticing that the angry response seems to stop them from moving forward in the situation.

These kinds of observations and interactions help to assess the state of a person's Wood Element. Given the negative feelings of a Wood type, what becomes important?

BIG ISSUES AND UNANSWERED QUESTIONS FOR THE WOOD TYPE

For any type, when typical negative experiences recur, certain issues become more important than others. The Big Issues for the Wood type are:

♦ Power
♦ Boundaries
♦ Correctness
♦ Growth
♦ Development

To say that these are Big Issues is to say that in any situation, particularly one of stress, the Wood type will almost automatically be concerned with who has the power or control, what are the boundaries, what is correct behaviour and how to develop and grow. Depending on the strategies the Wood type has chosen, some of these will be more important than others.

Another way of expressing the internal experience of someone whose Wood is constitutionally impaired is that they begin, to varying degrees, to carry certain unanswered questions such as:

♦ Why can't I have what I want?
♦ How should things be organized?
♦ Why am I blocked or stopped in this way?
♦ What do I really want?
♦ What is the point in trying when I know I cannot have it?

For the non-Wood type, there are answers to these questions. For the Wood type, these questions keep recurring, and to varying degrees do not get answered. The difficulty in finding answers to these questions can lead a Wood type to develop various life-patterns or strategies.

HOW WOULD YOU KNOW YOUR FRIEND IS A WOOD TYPE?

He or she might:

♦ have a greenish colour around the eyes
♦ speak with a clipped voice tone
♦ never get angry or suddenly get angry
♦ get angry at times when it would seem better not to
♦ have issues about the rules, boundaries and structures
♦ have a hard time making decisions
♦ have a directness about their gaze

RESPONSES TO THE BIG ISSUES

The ways of coping which we will discuss next are a response to the Big Issues and Unanswered Questions. Given that these issues are important and that the questions keep recurring, these are the kinds of life styles or behaviours which a Wood type might adopt to deal with their issues.

Not every Wood type will use all of these coping strategies and there may be other variations which we haven't observed. It is also possible for other types to behave in similar ways. In this case the behaviours might be less pronounced or have a different set of questions behind them.

The responses are:

♦ Organizing, structuring and getting things right
♦ Rebelling against the rules
♦ Seeking justice
♦ Indirectness
♦ Not planning or wanting anything

We will discuss each of these in turn.

Organizing, Structuring and Getting Things Right

Wood types can often be concerned about rules, structures and boundaries. Organizing and structuring are natural activities and most of the time they go unnoticed. A plan of what we're going to do for the day is a structure. We might consider what to wear, how to deal with traffic on the roads, how to prioritize our work, what to buy in the shops or what to eat for supper, all with very little effort. Dividing up the jobs when we go camping is structuring. Deciding how to organize our books on a new bookshelf is structuring. Sorting how we will run a meeting is structuring.

Wood types often have issues around organizing. This can manifest in their life as a keenness for organizing or the opposite, hating to structure, or both at different times. For example, the Wood type may in their personal life be very poor at structuring, but in their work really enjoy, and be good at it. Harry, a Wood type said:

I like to get everything sorted out and tidied up, whether it's the schedules for the week, the invoices sent out or the maintenance jobs to be done. I put everything up on the board and everybody knows exactly what has to be done by when. At home I'm quite different. I'm much more of a slob and I can have difficulty getting even the smallest jobs done.

Often Wood types who are good at organizing find it difficult when others are not as well structured as they are. They may especially like to see everything done in the correct way. Delia describes this:

I just challenge things — I pick up on things if they're not quite right. Things don't sit comfortably with me unless they're right and I get frustrated if they're not. I also expect it of myself and I'm my greatest critic. It might show as impatience. It's difficult to sit down and let someone else organize something as I know I can do it better.

Good organization helps people to know where they are. If an organization is not well structured this can create chaos. Lack of structure or things done badly can be especially unsettling for some Wood types who like things to be carried out correctly. For example, Julia told us:

I hate it when anybody breaks 'the rules'. I can never understand why people don't keep appointments on time or don't keep promises. I have a clear sense of what's right and I try to follow that. When someone else blatantly ignores what's right I feel frustrated.

Good structures and planning should make anything from an office, to a party, to an airport work better. Many Wood types can be found at the heart of an organization feeling literally 'in their Element' as they create well-organized administration. They can excel in creating clear rules and guidelines for others and setting up systems. As well as having a flair for administration, some of the many other jobs for good structurers could be as architects, town planners, air traffic controllers, accountants, teachers or designers.

At the other extreme some Wood types don't relate so easily to rules, structures and boundaries. Any constraints put on them may lead them to rebel.

Rebelling Against the Rules

The Wood Element gives us the ability to assert ourselves in the world. When it's imbalanced this natural inclination may become exaggerated. This can lead Wood types to push themselves forward more forcefully than other types. Any obstacle against this force may be kicked to one side. In some contexts this may be seen as rebellion.

Teenagers often rebel against the rules. This can enable them to find their own identity in order to separate from their parents and family. Jasmine, a Wood type, here recalls being rebellious:

> Historically I found boundaries difficult. I had very constraining parents and I had to break every rule. If I was asked not to do it, I'd do it or I became devious in order to break the rules. I didn't want to be controlled. I still often feel that way now.

Often Wood types find that they have an ambivalence about structures and boundaries. On the one hand they can love them because they know where they are with them. On the other hand they might find them constraining and want to push them away. Colin, who was in the fire service, explained this well:

I hate constraints being set up against me and I immediately rebel. In the fire service I chaffed against the rules and regulations. Then when I became an officer I thought — these aren't so bad after all.

When we adhere to good rules things flow more easily. On the other hand, some structures and conventions get out of date or are not productive and it does require confrontation and maybe even rebellion to change these. Social change is in part a record of these rebellions.

For many Wood types rebellion is their natural environment. If they do not have a worthwhile reason for rebelling, then they will rebel in any case and go for a change. In so doing, they change the distribution of space and we can often feel, from the outside, that our space has been taken up. Simon told us:

I have a lot of 'front'. I'm up front and talk to people and tell them what I want. I don't always give them much space. In fact I can be oblivious to them sometimes. I know if it was me I'd be livid.

Jacqueline also notices that she feels as if she takes up more space at times:

Sometimes I see myself as bigger than I am. I often feel that I rise to the occasion. I come over as being assertive and people get the impression that I am assertive. I pull out a confident front although I'm not necessarily at all confident.

The next pattern is in some ways an extension of 'being rebellious'.

Seeking Justice

Some Wood types use their excess energy and rebelliousness by protesting against things or by seeking justice for others. Their frustrations and anger then get positively channelled and become righteous indignation. Many Wood types hate to see injustice of any kind. Julie told us:

I abhor seeing people being badly treated. I also get angry about inequality. When I heard that company directors are getting huge pay rises I felt like spitting blood. What about all the poor people? Don't they care? I get frustrated because I can't do anything. I often write letters to my MP though. I get rid of some of my frustration that way.

Wood types will often join organizations which are aimed at making the world a better place. Rachel, for example, told us:

> I've been a member of Friends of the Earth and Greenpeace where meetings are full of people like myself who are protesting. We are always thinking of plans and ideas about how to improve the world. We feel strongly that if everybody took responsibility by not driving unnecessarily or by recycling their rubbish it would make the world a better place to live.

There are many ways that people can seek betterment for others. People can become MPs, local councillors, solicitors or barristers in order to fight for the rights for others. Others like Rachel may join organizations such as Greenpeace, Friends of the Earth or Amnesty International or they may take up lobbying. These Wood types may spotlight miscarriages of justice, lobby for animal rights, march for world peace or lobby for many other areas of social change or the rights of others.

Many other Wood types will fight quietly for the rights of their colleagues and friends when necessary. This may be at work via their union or just by standing up to the boss who is being short sighted in dealing with her or his employees. Not all the people who protest and lobby are Wood types of course but there will be a fair percentage of this type pursuing their feelings of indignation in good causes. Here a colleague described a Wood type she knows:

> I have a friend who always has an issue. He says, 'You've got to give it a shout. If you don't shout about it nothing gets done.' He goes to all the meetings, stands for elections and does anything to get in to say something in protest. Issues can be legalize cannabis, new roads, close circuit TV, anything that stops people from having freedom. He even sings protest songs and is a good musician!

We can speculate about the first singers of protest songs in the 60s and wonder if many of them were Wood types. Many of Bob Dylan's songs such as 'Masters of War' still ring loud in people's ears. We can also look at many other well-known protesters such as Martin Luther King who started the civil rights movement in the US when he was appalled by the lack of rights for black people. Christabel Pankhurst, who we write about at the end of this chapter, fought tirelessly to gain women the right to vote and Elizabeth Fry worked to reform British prisons in the last century.

The next pattern is less up front than 'seeking justice'.

Indirectness

We are all indirect at times and this is appropriate. When we are direct, we are aware of our own desires and are willing to 'own' these desires publicly. This enables us, when necessary, to ask for what we want. Some Wood types find this difficult. Often they are reacting to the past. They may have been prevented from getting what they wanted at an earlier stage of their lives. Subsequently they compensated by becoming indirect.

In order to understand this better we can go back to the child who is reaching for a toy and is told 'No!' Soon the child anticipates the 'No'. She begins to check if the preventing parent is present. This is perhaps using natural caution. The caution later becomes internalized so that the child proceeds more and more indirectly. For example, the child may say to her parent, 'My friend Billy (and by implication not me) likes to play with this toy.' As time goes on the Wood type may stop owning their natural desires. They may still ask for things, but indirectly.

At times being indirect can be useful. We may know what we want but understand that it is best not to state this publicly. Sometimes, for example, it may be the best way to move forward. Challenging people head on is not always a good idea. Eleanor has to deal with some angry customers at the travel company where she works. She told us:

> Sometimes people complain about their holidays and they're almost wanting to pick a fight. I have to do my best to diffuse the situation to avoid a head-on confrontation. It can be difficult and I often have to suppress my own feelings to do it.

Another Wood type, who is a friend of ours, uses her chronic inability to be direct in a positive way. She is a hypnotherapist and has become very skilled at making indirect and useful suggestions which enable her clients to make positive changes in their lives.

Many Wood types can swing between being very direct and indirect. If we avoid being direct too much we may feel a need to take it out on other people. As Eleanor told us:

> At work, if someone criticizes me I'll avoid dealing with the situation at all costs. I'll try and pretend that I haven't noticed. It will affect me though and

later on I know I often go on a 'go slow' with my work. I suppose it's my way of paying them back.

Being indirect can also manifest in our sense of humour as Jacqueline admitted:

If I can't be directly angry I can sometimes find myself making bitchy remarks. I've got a nasty cutting edge to my humour and I realize I've sometimes offended people deeply.

At the worst extreme we may not be able to be direct with ourselves. In this case we may end up losing touch with ourselves and what we want. Excessive indirectness can lead to an apparent absence of desires.

Not Planning or Wanting Anything

Sometimes the ability to assert ourselves in the world seems missing. Wood types like this often don't have a strong notion of what they want.

In these circumstances the missing part is usually supplied from without. The Wood type may find someone to replace their capacity to set boundaries, create structures and define who they are. For example, joining a cult, enlisting in the army or perhaps marrying a dominating person may replace their self-determination. The cult, the army or the other person gives them a purpose, and makes many of their decisions for them. Colin, who we spoke to earlier in the chapter, could understand this:

I find the idea of being in the armed forces appealing and can relate to those who join. It's the routine and the structure and knowing what's expected of me. It's knowing where I am with it.

Simon knows he finds external structure helpful and purposely brings it into his life:

I like structures imposed to some extent because then I have to do things. I know I can make things happen but I don't do a lot to make them — it's easier not to. I know I could easily drift and I don't want to. I choose people who are well-organized to be around me. My last flatmate for example was very strong on boundaries and I value that and appreciate our different qualities.

At the extreme, people without internal structure may not know what they want. In this case they may be so adaptable and take on an outside structure so easily that they either play into the hands of others or cause others to feel frustrated. In the former case, the outsider has found a compliant and useful helper; in the latter, the outsider knows something is not quite right, but doesn't know what it is. Paul told us:

Whatever happens is OK with me. I don't need a big career or somewhere I'm going. I am just happy to be. I am not asking for anything.

When the pattern is extreme, a person has no life plan and their 'Hun', which we mentioned earlier, is not manifesting in the world. This position sounds attractive and can even masquerade as a form of spirituality — truly just Being with no compulsion to do anything in order to achieve results. It can also result in no work, limited possessions and minimal relationships which is not an easy position to maintain for long.

This 'not apparently wanting anything' is an inability to assert ourselves in the world — which is the capacity of the Wood Element.

VIRTUES AND VICES OF A WOOD TYPE

Depending on the health of the Wood type, these ways of coping produce both virtues and vices. Some of the virtues are:
♦ a strong capacity to organize
♦ a commitment to continuous growth
♦ a capacity for determining rightness or correctness and a resolve to see this carried out with justice
♦ a useful warrior mentality
♦ a youthfulness, even in old age, born out of a commitment to continue growing.
    Some of the vices are:
♦ over-attention to structuring, detail and rules
♦ over-assertive behaviour which can lead to chronic belligerence
♦ repetitive rebellion which forgets the outcome of growth or development
♦ never admitting to the real goals and ends
♦ passive stuckness which has forgotten the real ends.

A FAMOUS WOOD TYPE — CHRISTABEL PANKHURST[6]

Wood type Christabel Pankhurst was born in 1880. Along with her mother Emmeline and her sister Sylvia, she is famous for her militant crusade which culminated in women gaining the right to vote. She had a combination of many of the Wood type strategies mentioned above. Like many Wood types she was a 'justice seeker' and channelled her assertion into positive rebellion, challenging the rules in order to create social change. She was also a natural 'structurer' and was known to be a formidable organizer. Her belief in 'getting things right' led her to achieve her aims with one-pointed directness.

As a child, Christabel was brought up in an atmosphere of revolution. Her father passionately believed in fighting for women's rights. Christabel's own fight intensified, however, when on deciding to enter the legal profession she found to her anger and dismay that the profession was barred to women.

In 1903, Christabel along with Emmeline and Sylvia, formed the Women's Social and Political Union (WSPU). From then on Christabel used an increasingly militant campaign to lobby for the vote. As well as being an impressive organizer, she was also a gifted orator. Her Wood type personality helped her to argue the case for women's suffrage by speaking all over the country. When speaking to many women's groups she roused many other women to give up their jobs and dedicate themselves to the cause.

Of the two sisters, Christabel and Sylvia, Christabel was the most forceful. Sylvia noted that her sister became more autocratic in her leadership style as time went on. She started her campaign by unceasingly challenging every politician she met. Over the years, however, she increased her militancy, making sure she was arrested and imprisoned for 'assaulting' a policeman and later on by inciting suffragettes to go on hunger strike and chaining themselves to public buildings. She is quoted as saying about the organization she formed:

The WSPU is a fighting organization, it must have one policy, one movement and one command.

It was only during the first world war that she stopped campaigning and put all of her energy into the war effort.

The fight for votes for women was finally won in 1918, after the First World War. It was seen that women could work as long and hard as any man. Women over 30 were given the vote. It wasn't until 1928, however, that women were given the right to vote at the same age as men.

After 1918 Christabel had no cause to follow and nowhere to channel her rebellious spirit and anger. She tried to get elected to parliament and failed. She then became a revivalist and toured America, lecturing about the second coming of Christ. She used the same fervent energy as a revivalist as she had used as a suffragette. She divided her time between Britain and the US and made money from her lectures and the books she wrote. She finally died in 1958.

SOME GOLDEN RULES FOR WOOD TYPES

♦ Knowing the rules, structures and boundaries is important.
♦ Rules, boundaries and structures are sometimes your choice, sometimes others' and sometimes shared.
♦ Your growth and development is smoother if you take responsibility for the rules, boundaries and structures you accept and create.
♦ Put your higher values into the world.
♦ It is often useful to check with others where they are coming from and what are their higher values compared to yours.

Notes

1   A description of the characters for the Elements can be found in Weiger, L, 1965: *Chinese Characters.*

2   The Organ functions are described in terms of 'Qi' and 'Blood'. These are also terms specific to Chinese medicine. The Chinese term for energy is 'Qi' (pronounced chee) which has many meanings depending upon individual contexts. In its widest use, 'Qi' is the underlying energy of the body-mind. So, for example, some Organs are more important for creating new Qi, e.g. the Stomach, and some are more important for keeping the Qi flowing smoothly, e.g. the Liver. The Chinese notion of 'Blood' overlaps considerably with our Western understanding. The functions of 'Blood' in Chinese medicine are to nourish, moisten and provide a 'root' for the mind. The notion of a root for the mind will be briefly explained in the chapter on the Fire type. Anyone wanting to discover more about the concepts of Chinese medicine is referred to: Hicks, John: *The Principles of Chinese Herbal Medicine* or Hicks, Angela: *The Principles of Chinese Medicine* and *The Principles of Acupuncture.*

3   These metaphorical descriptions were given in the Nei Jing referred to in Note
    4, Chapter 1. A source of these where the relevant chapter of the Nei Jing is
    translated and commented upon is: Larre, Claude and Rochat de la Vallee,
    Elisabeth (trans), 1987: *The Secret Treatise of the Spiritual Orchid*. They can be
    found in a briefer form in Chapter 8 of Maoshing Ni (trans), 1995: *The Yellow
    Emperor's Classic of Medicine*.

4   'The Effects of Anger on Left Ventricular Fraction in Coronary Artery Disease'
    by Gail Ironson et al. Published in the *American Journal of Cardiology* in 1992.
    Pages 281–285.

5   Daniel Goleman: *Emotional Intelligence*; Bloomsbury Publishing, Chapter 11,
    page 170.

6   The information in this section is taken from: Castle, Barbara, 1987: *Sylvia and
    Christabel Pankhurst*.

Chapter 3

EXERCISES FOR WOOD TYPES

INTRODUCTION

The exercises in this section are aimed at enabling Wood types to find a better emotional balance. Some useful goals for Wood types are:

♦ To become more conscious of the motives and purposes behind their everyday activities
♦ To be able to get in touch with their deeper wishes in order to evaluate everyday situations
♦ To 'own' and become more expressive about their deeper wants or desires
♦ To learn to negotiate with others so that everyone gains, thereby creating win/win interactions
♦ To formulate more satisfying long and short term goals.

USING THE EXERCISES

We suggest that you read an exercise through before you start it. All of the exercises are laid out in a similar style. Following the *introduction*, we tell you approximately *how long* it will take to complete. Obviously some of you will take more time and others less. The exercises are then divided into stages. They start with:

♦ the *purpose* of the exercise and then
♦ the *process* or the steps of the exercise.

The theme of each step is in bold so that you have a summary. At the end of some exercises we have a section called *'matters arising'*. Here we discuss issues which could come up while you do the exercise.

THE EXERCISES FOR WOOD TYPES

- ♦ Focusing
- ♦ The other person's point of view
- ♦ The objective point of view
- ♦ Finding what I *really* want
- ♦ Forgiveness
- ♦ Protecting ourselves
- ♦ Understanding the other person
- ♦ Enacting forgiveness
- ♦ Beating cushions
- ♦ A Qigong exercise for the Liver

EXERCISE 1 — FOCUSING

Introduction

Dave was frequently feeling, as he said, 'frustrated' in office meetings. The feelings he had made him less effective in the meeting and uncomfortable afterwards, sometimes for days. He tried the exercise below called 'Focusing'. Through the exercise he discovered that his 'frustration' had two parts. One was that his mind was often ahead of the group and the second was that he felt the others did not give him any credit for his contributions. The feelings changed and he felt more comfortable, which led him to find different ways to express himself in meetings.
Time needed: Anything from 10 to 20 minutes or more.

Purpose

This exercise helps us to clarify what we are feeling. As our emotions are made up of parts, we do not always know exactly what we are feeling.[1]

Process

Focusing can be applied to unclear feelings, an unclear situation or thoughts which are not understood. The exercise below is written as if you have not pinpointed which of these to start with. If you already know where you are starting begin with step 3.

1 **Scan for the Issues.** Find a quiet, comfortable place to do the exercise. Scan through your body paying attention to how you feel inside. Notice any feelings of discomfort or thoughts which are nagging you unpleasantly.

If nothing comes up, you can ask yourself, 'Why don't I feel wonderful right now?' and wait for an answer. (Of course, if you do feel wonderful, you might want to forget this exercise!) Often you can make a list which might look like:
   ◆ an uncomfortable tightness down my chest
   ◆ the 'issue I have with George'
   ◆ the feeling in my lower abdomen which I think is linked to a discussion about money with my partner
   ◆ a vague achy feeling just above my eyes.

2 **Pick an Issue**. Decide on which feeling, situation or thought is the most important to you. If you can't decide, just pick one.

3 **Get a 'felt sense' of the problem as a whole.** Do not enter into the feelings so much as simply get a 'sense' of them. This can be called a 'felt sense' which is a 'holistic, unclear sense of the whole thing'. As this process is for dealing with something which is unclear, you may need to try this out for a while before you think you know what you are doing.

4 **Find a Handle.** Find a word, phrase or image which represents the core of the 'felt sense' of the problem. Let this come from the 'felt sense'. This may take some time and a good degree of concentration – give it whatever it needs. Various words or pictures will come up until, with one, you will just feel 'that's right'. At the same time the 'felt sense' may change a bit. Examples of handles are:
   ◆ 'shamed'
   ◆ 'stuck'
   ◆ 'heavy and impenetrable'
   ◆ a picture of a tree being chopped down
   ◆ a dark image of a sphere with light coming out from below.

5   **Resonate back and forth** between the word, phrase or image and the 'felt sense'. Your purpose is to check the rightness of the 'fit' between the word, phrase or image and the 'felt sense'. It is good if you feel some releasing of energy and the 'felt sense' may change somewhat.

6   **Asking.** Now pay attention directly to the 'felt sense'. Ask 'What is it about the whole issue which is X?', where X is the word, phrase or image. Using the examples above, the questions to ask might be: 'What is it about the whole issue which is shamed or shameful?'

Now wait for the answer. Allow it to come from the 'felt sense' rather than from your mind. Answers which come fast are often from the mind. These have no impact on the felt sense. An answer which comes from the felt sense may take longer to come and often also creates a mental or physical 'shift'. Often they give us a new perspective on ourselves or our feelings. We do not control when a shift comes. So just wait.

Here are two other questions which you might ask. Over time you might find others.

♦ What does the felt sense need?

♦ What is the worst of this?

Ask. Wait for the body shift. Do not presume that you know or can judge what will happen. You started on the assumption that you did not know.

7   **Receiving.** Whatever body shifts you get, just receive them. They may turn into words and you may not agree with them, but just receive them. Re-ask and more shifts may occur. Know that you may have achieved a partial shift and more will arise. Another way of continuing is to recycle through the previous steps.

8   **Finishing.** When you wish to finish the session it is best to do so gently. There are some times in this process when there is more activity and other times when there is less. Allow your body to tell you when it is at a resting period and it is a good time to stop. If you want to explore more later on, it is often useful to tell the part you have been in contact with that you will be back.

EXERCISE 2 — THE OTHER'S POINT OF VIEW

Introduction

In an earlier example, Dave used 'Focusing' to clarify his feelings of frustration which arose in meetings. One thing he did after this discovery was to step into the shoes of several of his colleagues. He discovered that they were probably experiencing him as angry — which surprised him — and he speculated that if they did, this might explain why they seemed unfriendly and did not give him the credit he expected.

Time needed: 10–20 minutes. Later you will be able to do this more quickly in any situation.

Purpose

The purpose of this exercise is to experience the world from the point of view of another person. The exercise is usually practised with respect to someone you have interacted with often and might be in conflict with. It is intended to bring information which is relevant, but which you might not otherwise have noticed.

Process

1 **Pick a person you wish to understand.** Think of someone you are in contact with, possibly with difficulty and perhaps in conflict. Find a specific moment in time when you were with them.
2 **Find a purpose for doing the exercise.** For example, you may want to:
   ♦ understand why they responded to you in a certain way
   ♦ stay in rapport with them
   ♦ understand what they will do next or
   ♦ know what it will be like to work with them.
3 **Get a sense of the person.** In your imagination see the other person in front of you and notice her or his breathing, posture, facial expression, gestures and voice tone. Remember other important areas which might relate to your situation with the person. These might include their age, experience, abilities, health, problems, relationships and needs.
4 **Step into the other person's point of view.** Imagine you are that person and can feel as she or he feels. You may find it easiest to actually change

positions as you become the other person. As the other person, see what they are seeing at the time, hear what they hear and feel any emotions involved.

Gently ask yourself how does this person experience me? It might be useful to use the other person's name. For example, if your name is Susan and the person whose shoes you are going to wear is Pete, then you can say to yourself to aid the identification, 'I am Pete and I am looking at Susan.'

You may find that you can do this task immediately or it may take you a while. If it takes time, remind yourself that you are developing a very useful skill and persist.

5 **Gather relevant information.** Once you are in the other person's place, and not before, gather information relevant to your purpose. If you want to know how the person feels about you, describe to yourself as Pete, how you are feeling about Susan. If you want Pete to trust you more, ask yourself, as Pete, whether you trust Susan and if not, why not. Other questions you might ask are:

♦ What do I want?

♦ How do I feel?

♦ What am I thinking?

♦ What would change things for me right now?

6 **Come back into yourself.** Some people do this activity so well that they need to, literally, shake off how the other person is feeling. Those who easily take on another person, however, are less likely to need to do this exercise! Other people easily come back to themselves. If necessary stand up and shake yourself and then pay careful attention to note that you are back to normal.

EXERCISE 3 — THE OBJECTIVE POINT OF VIEW

Introduction

Brenda had two teenage sons and was not happy with the way she was relating to them. From the previous exercise — the other person's point of view — she discovered that her sons were different and that both were changing in their feelings towards her. She needed some new understanding of how to relate to them. The following exercises gave her the insights she needed. She continued periodically to use this exercise with respect to the boys and says the results helped her to understand many of their needs as they developed into adults.

Time needed: At first, 10 minutes to half an hour. Later you will be much quicker.

Purpose

This exercise enables us to experience things from an objective point of view, which is sometimes called the perspective of the 'neutral observer' or even the 'wise person'.

Process

1 **Pick a person or situation you wish to understand.** This may be a difficulty which is not turning out as you want it to, or a person you don't understand. It is best if some new insights or perceptions would be useful.
2 **Prepare some helpful questions.** (These assume that your name is Susan and the other person is called Pete). The following are just examples:
   ♦ What does Susan (you) want and what does Pete (the other significant person) really want?
   ♦ What is going on between these two?
   ♦ What is stopping progress?
   ♦ Is there something Susan does not know but should?
   ♦ Would a change of attitude help?
   ♦ What is the best way for Susan to act?
3 **Put yourself in the objective point of view.** Find a comfortable place where you know you will not be disturbed. Imagine a typical situation in which you find yourself and the other person. See the situation from the point of view of a neutral observer and imagine that you are watching both yourself and the other person.

   You may find it easiest to actually change positions as you do this exercise. In this case you may wish to place yourself and the other person on two chairs in front of you. Sit on a third chair watching them.
4 **Now adjust your perspective:** Notice the people in your image. Adjust them so that they are similar in size, distance and clarity. If there are any voices adjust them so that they come from the person who is speaking.

   If your pictures don't seem clear, don't worry. It is more important that you have a *sense* of the people involved and that the scene displays the characters equally. It is best to refer to each person in the scene by their names or by the pronouns 'he' or 'she'. If you are Susan and the other person in the scene is Pete, you may say, 'Susan is over there and Pete is over there. She is wearing ... and he is wearing ...'.

Your adjustment of the image so far is designed to develop your capacity for objectivity. You may achieve it the first time — it may well take longer.

5 **Ask the questions you have prepared.** Set up the modified scene and as you hold it in mind, ask the questions you prepared. Take whatever time you need. Notice from your objective position both what the other person is saying and doing and also how you are responding.

6 **Notice any changes in your original feelings.** Go back to your original feelings and notice if you feel any differently about them. If you get any useful information, you may wish to write it down. You may have found new ways of dealing with the situation.

Matters Arising

Some people may find that they do this exercise easily. For others it takes practice to set up the scene properly and to hold it while you ask the questions and receive the answers. You may decide to set up a practice programme, for example, once a day for two weeks until you are fluent. It may take a short time and it may take longer. Keep the potential benefits in mind.

EXERCISE 4 — FINDING WHAT I *REALLY* WANT

Introduction

Dennis used this exercise to make himself more effective in his meetings and in his whole work situation. By discovering what was really important to him and comparing this with what was important to others, he felt that he had clarified his 'work-landscape' considerably. He certainly became a more effective part of the team by clarifying his own values or higher purposes.

Time needed: 15–30 minutes.

Purpose

This exercise is about answering that all important question: 'What do I really want?' It helps us to answer the question, not just in terms of immediate and physical goals, but also in terms of our higher purposes. Rather than just thinking 'I want a job', 'I want a nice home', or 'I want to be promoted', this exercise helps us determine the reasons or purposes behind these goals. Knowing these can give us much more flexibility and integrate the everyday world of physical objects with our higher purpose, which is both more internal and external.

Process

1 **Pick an area of your life you wish to work on.** In this case it can be:
   ♦ A circumstance you are in with someone else — especially where there is some conflict
   ♦ A part of your life — like your work, relationship, leisure or parenting
   ♦ Any activity you engage in which takes your time and interest
   ♦ In the widest sense — life itself.

2 **Keeping this area in mind, ask yourself 'What is important here?'** The answers you come up with should be standards or values rather than behaviours.

   Let's use an example. Jane has chosen to examine her work where she is often in conflict within a committee. Jane and a work colleague are approaching the problem quite differently. When Jane asks herself 'What is important here?' she answers, taking time and going inside for the answers:
   ♦ achieving the goals of the organization
   ♦ mutual understanding
   ♦ preserving standards
   ♦ keeping the good will of the team
   ♦ enjoying my work
   ♦ getting credit for what I have done.

   We can say that these are the values that Jane would apply to this area. Values are often expressed in a single word or phrase, e.g. 'fun', 'satisfaction', 'honesty', 'love', 'a sense of rightness', or 'doing things elegantly'. They usually arise quite easily in response to the question 'What is important about ...?'

3 **Continue to process the values.** There are two ways to do this. Process your set of values in both ways.

   First find the values behind the values:
   ♦ 'If I could achieve ... what is important about that?' By asking this question you are uncovering the values which lie behind the original value. Carry on generating more values by asking the question over again. At a certain place you may find no more answers and you have found your highest value.

   Jane, for example, might ask, 'If I could achieve *preserving standards* what would be important about that?' Her answer might be 'job satisfaction'. She then asks, 'If I could achieve *job satisfaction* what would be important about that?' She continues to ask herself the question until she has found her highest value.

Now prioritize your values:

♦ List your values and put the most important at the top, the second most important second, and so on. This can take some time and you may discover that one value supports another. For instance, Jane might realize that 'mutual understanding' usually leads to 'enjoying my work' and that is why it is important.

4   **Consider the area you have worked on and whether your values are being achieved.** For example, if we consider the work context and the specific committee, Jane might ask the following questions:

♦ In that context, am I achieving my values?

♦ When I consider a specific situation of conflict, does having clarity about my values help me resolve the conflict? For example, does it make it easier for me to compromise because I know which values are most important to me? If not,

♦ Do others share my values and would a discussion about values be useful?

   If you have truly specified your values and you begin to achieve them, you are on the way to satisfaction or at least doing and achieving what is really important to you.

5   **Do this with several areas and update yourself frequently.** As suggested above, you will benefit from finding your values and hence becoming clear about what is important for you. Later you may wish to update your values and it is useful to see which of your values remain constant and which change.

Matters Arising

You might make discoveries about changes you need to make in the area you worked on. For instance, in the work context if 'getting paid' is your lowest value or not even on the list, it may explain why you are having a problem paying your bills. If, in the relationship context, where you are parenting and sharing a heavy work load, 'fun and having a good time' is your highest value, you will definitely need to be creative or at least learn how to make light of changing nappies.

Usually when values emerge and you stand back and look at them, these kinds of insights pop up. It might be interesting to compare the values of your partner and yourself — remember that argument we had last week ...?

As it is important to do this exercise several times, choose one area now but over a period of time expect to cover different ones. Some might overlap — like 'work' and 'a situation where you are in conflict with someone'.

EXERCISE 5 — FORGIVENESS[2]

Introduction

At work, Penny had a colleague who had once deliberately misled her when they were both going for the same job. They ended up working on the same project and frequently have to cooperate. Penny held a grudge against this colleague and her feelings interfered with the working relationship and frequently left Penny feeling uncomfortable. Penny used the following exercise to 'forgive' her colleague. She did not end up trusting that the colleague never would mislead her again, but she did feel accepting of the person and comfortable working together. Penny was not aware of how much our health can be eroded by carrying around resentment, but she said in retrospect, that this seemed a much more human way to behave.

Bearing grudges and remaining resentful are dangerous to our health. We often continue resentment for two reasons. One is that we do not want to give up the one indicator — in the form of our anger, bitterness or grudge — that whatever was done to us was unacceptable. The other is a feeling that our forgiveness might allow the other person to abuse or violate us again in a similar way. So the exercise is broken into three stages:

- ♦ The first deals with the objections we have about being a pushover and inviting more of the same treatment. We call this one 'Protecting Ourselves'.
- ♦ The second attempts to understand the person with whom we are still angry. If we can achieve some understanding, it is easier to let go of the anger itself. We call this one 'Understanding the Other Person'.
- ♦ The third is to actually forgive and feel different. This involves thinking about the other person in the same way that we think about the others we have forgiven. We call this one 'Enacting Forgiveness'. You can do these in three sittings or in one go.

EXERCISE 5a — PROTECTING OURSELVES

Purpose

The purpose of this stage is to protect ourselves from any further abuse or violation, especially from the person in question.
Time needed: 5–10 minutes

Process

1 **Describe who and what causes you still to be angry.** Write down the names of people against whom you are holding resentment. Take small incidents if you do not have big ones. Describe what you felt was violated. You can include both physical trauma and your internal values. The kind of things people say are:

   ♦ My head and sides were kicked; I took three weeks to recover, and I realized that I was left with an ongoing low-grade feeling of fear. I believe it is wrong to get drunk and take out your grievances on someone random.

   ♦ Those twisting words made me doubt myself. It is not fair to manipulate someone in that way.

   ♦ He threatened my child and I felt helpless. I think it's unfair to get at me through my child.

   ♦ I did so much for her and she repaid me with betrayal. Accepting from someone and doing the dirty behind their back is not on.

2 **Clarify how you can protect yourself from similar abuse.** You may stay away from the person, but you may need to encounter them because of your circumstances. For example, if you continue attending college or working in the same office. It may be helpful to ask other people how they would protect themselves.

   There is often a trade-off here that we hesitate to make. We 'need' to attend work, but that puts us in a vulnerable position. We might actually like the person in some ways or we may even feel sorry for them. At the same time we may be worried that our contact with her or him may expose us to a similar violation. Use exercise number 3 above, the Objective Point of View, and at stage 5 ask yourself how, realistically, you can protect yourself. Act on the information you receive.

EXERCISE 5b — UNDERSTANDING THE OTHER PERSON

Purpose

The purpose of this stage is to understand more about the person who violated or offended you.

Time needed: 15–30 minutes.

Process

1 **Go to the 'Other's point of view'.** (See Exercise 2 above). Go to the position of the other person and ask yourself what was important about doing whatever you (the other person) did. You are asking about their intentions or values and you may get answers which are very different from those you would give. Keep asking this question until you receive an answer to which you could say, 'Yes, I can accept this as a reason, even though the behaviour is not acceptable.' For the difference between behaviour and the underlying intention see 'Matters Arising' below.

2 **Consider what education, training or resources the other person might have had that would enable her or him to behave differently.** When you have some idea about this, go to Exercise 3 to find the objective point of view again. Go through the time you were violated or abused but imagining how the other would have behaved had they had different education, training or resources.

Matters Arising

A useful belief which comes from Neuro Linguistic Programming is that people may behave badly but underlying this is a 'positive intention'.[3] For example, the positive intention of people who have injured others could be that they wished to have a 'bit of fun with their friends'. The behaviour is *unacceptable*, the outcome or intention may be *acceptable* and the person is very *short on resources*. Resources in this sense are the education, training or skills which will enable the person to achieve 'a bit of fun with their friends' in a variety of ways, and without injuring others.

It can be important to remember that all of us at one time or another try to satisfy our own reasonable needs and, through ignorance, injure others. This awareness does not in any way condone or pardon the behaviour.

EXERCISE 5c — ENACTING FORGIVENESS

Purpose

The purpose of this stage is to let go of the negative feelings associated with the person who abused or violated you.
Time needed: 20–30 minutes.

Process

1 **Check whether you still harbour the grudge.** Remind yourself that you have taken steps to protect yourself. You have also gained at least some understanding of the other person's behaviour. If you are free of the negative feelings, and you may well be, then the exercise is over. Congratulations for letting go of feelings that would have harmed you! If the feelings are still there, then proceed with the rest of this exercise.

2 **Find a person who has made you temporarily angry,** *but you quickly forgave*. This should be a person that briefly made you angry or irritated, but *never* caused you to harbour a grudge. You may now even think of her or him with compassion or good feeling. In your mind's eye imagine this person is in front of you. Notice your image of the person and check the following areas:
   ♦ What is the size, location, distance and clarity of your image?
   ♦ Is the person in the picture moving or still?
   ♦ Is there a frame around the picture or is it open-ended?
   ♦ Is it coloured or black and white?
   ♦ Are there any sounds or voices and if so where do they come from?
   Jot down notes about how you represent the person. For instance, the picture may be life-sized, about three feet away, in clear focus and slightly to your right. The person could be moving slightly and the picture may be a bright colour. There may be a few words spoken by the person in the picture.

3 **Now think about the person for whom you harbour a grudge.** As in stage 2, in your mind's eye imagine that this person is in front of you. Notice your image of this person and check the following areas:
   ♦ What is the size, location, distance and clarity of your image?
   ♦ Is the person in the picture moving or still?
   ♦ Is there a frame around the picture or is it open-ended?
   ♦ Is it coloured or black and white?

♦ Are there any sounds or voices and if so where do they come from?

Jot down notes on how you represent this person. It will probably be different from the person in stage 2. For instance, the picture of the person who you resent might be smaller than the previous one, further away, slightly out of focus and to your left. She or he may not be moving and the picture may be in black and white with an unfocused frame around it. There may be no sound coming from the picture.

4   **Now, put the person for whom you harbour a grudge into the position and format of the person you easily forgave.** First, move the person to the same position. Then change the size, clarity, location, distance, colour, movement and sounds. This may take a moment or two to carry out.

We will use the example of the two people above, to demonstrate. This means that to put the person for whom we harbour a grudge, into the position and format of the person we easily forgave we carry out a number of steps. First, we would move the picture of the person we resented into the position held by the person we forgave. In the example this is from the left to the right. We could now change the picture to one which is life-sized, closer, brighter in colour, has movement in it and some sounds. It would now match the qualities of the picture of the person we forgave.

Hold the person you have resented in the position and format of the person you have forgiven. Notice if you can think about her or him in the same way as the person you have forgiven.

5   **Check to see if you can now think about that person without the negative feelings you had before**. If you have achieved this, congratulations. If you have not, then consider going back to exercises 5a and 5b, before cycling through this exercise again.

EXERCISE 6 — BEATING CUSHIONS

Introduction

Gerry once returned home from work, thinking he felt fine. He could not settle and realized that he had an uncomfortable feeling under his ribs and without it he knew he would feel much better. He thought of 'Focusing', but decided to try 'Beating cushions'. In the middle of beating, he was surprised at the strength of feeling that emerged and the words that came out of his mouth. It seemed to have needed the physical action to release this feeling. He was grateful for the insight and relief he achieved.

Time needed: 5–20 minutes.

Purpose

This exercise is a way of safely letting go of our blocked or stuck feelings. Sometimes these feelings develop into physical and mental symptoms such as headaches, muscle tensions, eye problems or the inability to plan ahead. Because these stuck feelings are often imploded anger, the exercises uses strong physical movement safely expressed.

Process

1 **Find a large pillow or mattress or something you can beat or use as a punch bag.** Find a quiet space where you won't be disturbed or bothered for at least half an hour. It helps for the second stage if it is fairly soundproof too! If you do not have this kind of space in your own house, if possible, ask a friend if you can use theirs. You may wish to have a trusted friend with you while you do this but *never* do it in the presence of a person with whom you don't feel safe.

2 **Place the cushion or mattress on the floor and kneel in front of it. Make a fist with your arms above your head. Bring them down on the cushion. Repeat in order to beat in a rhythmic movement.** As you beat the cushion you might find that you remember a situation or event from the past which you still feel angry about. Allow yourself to express the angry feelings that you had at the time by punching or beating the cushions. If you do not remember any situations or events just keep punching to release your angry feelings.

This may be enough for you to do in one session. You may find that punching the cushion releases a lot of your pent-up feelings.

3 **Now try shouting as you beat.** You might do this in the first session or at a later session. If you remember a situation that has made you angry find a short sentence which expresses what you want to say. This may be, 'Get lost!' or 'How dare you!' or just plain 'No!'. You can use stronger language to get the feelings out of your system if you wish.

4 **Keep shouting the same words over and over again in rhythm with your punching.** After a while you may decide to change to another sentence.

Continue beating and shouting. You may carry on for 10—20 minutes although some people may take a longer or shorter time. At a certain point you will feel finished for this session. You may feel that all of your anger has come out or that only some of your emotions have been released. You will often know when you have completely cleared your angry feelings, as good feelings then start to emerge.

5 **You may wish to do a small amount of cushion beating every day** — about ten minutes may be enough or you can do this for a longer period.

Matters Arising

Remember: clearing emotions can be an important release, but they will recur unless you also deal with the underlying causes. For example, we can be angry for many reasons. These can include not feeling appreciated, feeling frightened, not feeling respected or feeling unloved. Forgiveness (see previous exercise), for example, can be an essential ingredient for resolving anger — otherwise it may never be fully cleared.

If we find it difficult to beat cushions there are many other activities which can help us to release pent up angry feelings. This can include going for a run or a vigorous walk, playing tennis or other racquet games, skipping, jumping up and down, stamping the feet or banging on drums.

QIGONG EXERCISE FOR THE LIVER

Purpose

Wood types may tense up when they feel frustrated or angry and can feel especially tight around the area of the ribcage where the Liver and Gall Bladder lie. This exercise will loosen up this area and also stretch the channels of the Gall Bladder and Liver which travel down the sides.

Time needed: About 5 minutes a day.

Process

1 **Stand with your feet shoulder width apart and your knees slightly bent.** Keep the inside edges of your feet parallel. From your hips, bounce gently up and down. Feel how your weight travels down from your hips to your feet which are solid on the floor. Tuck your tailbone in so that your lower back is

straight. Draw your chin in slightly so that your spine stretches upward. Relax your chest and let the front of your abdomen drop.

2 **Now raise your arms above your head and lock your fingers together with your palms facing downwards.** This forms an arch over your head. Take a deep breath in, then breathe out.

3 **On the out breath gently rock to one side** and feel the stretch all the way down the opposite side of your body — on your arm, neck, ribs and down the side of your leg. Stay in this position for a few seconds, relaxing as you stretch.

4 **Now come back to the centre.** Breathe in again, then breathe out and repeat the exercise on the opposite side.

5 **Repeat this exercise,** 6 times on either side. (See Figure 3 below).

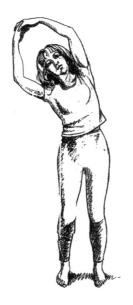

Figure 3: QIGONG EXERCISE FOR THE LIVER

Notes

1   See Gendlin, Eugene T, 1978: *Focusing*; Bantam Books, New York. Gendlin was a therapist who wondered why therapy worked some times and not others. After much research he believed it was the individual's ability to clarify their own feelings that made therapy work. He then devised the basic focusing exercise which we have adapted. See also Cornell, Ann Weiser, Ph.d.: *The Power of Focusing;* New Harbinger Publications.

2   In writing 'the forgiveness exercise' we have been helped by Andreas, Steve, 1991: *The Forgiveness Pattern* (audio tape); NLP Comprehensive, Boulder, Colorado.

3   For an excellent discussion of 'positive intention' and its role in understanding another person refer to Andreas, Connirae and Andreas, Steve, 1989: *Heart of the Mind*; Chapter 8.

Chapter 4

THE FIRE TYPE - LOVING OURSELVES

NADINE IS A FIRE TYPE

'When I realized I was a Fire type everything clicked into place', Nadine told us. 'I realized why I get hurt so easily — the slightest cross word, or disapproving look and I take it personally. It might not even be aimed at me but I immediately think people don't like me. The hurt goes right inside. The surprising thing is that on other days I can feel really bright and cheerful. On a good day I can bring the best out in people and cheer them up.'

As we got to know Nadine better she told us more about herself. 'On the surface I appear to be open to anybody, but it takes me a long time to really trust people enough to tell them what really matters to me. The truth is that I think people will reject me once they know the real me. Sometimes people think I'm flippant and that upsets me. I might sometimes make a joke when the mood gets serious but deep inside I really care about the world. I just don't always show it.'

Nadine's facial colour is pale and her emotions alternate between joy and sadness. She laughs a lot. Her understanding and insight allowed her to work on herself, especially around the area of her relationships which have often caused her problems. Although she is employed as a secretary, her boss regards her as a special asset because she can instantly relate to visitors and put them at ease. Although it is outside her job description, he often uses her to interview prospective employees because he values her insight.

As we look at the characteristics of Fire types throughout this chapter, it will become clearer why Nadine is a Fire type. We begin by examining the Fire Element in Chinese medicine.

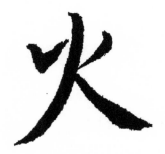

Figure 4: THE CHINESE CHARACTER FOR FIRE

THE FIRE ELEMENT IN NATURE

The Chinese character for Fire is Huo (see above) which signifies dancing or ascending flames.

A fire is hot, bright, vital and even radiant. We may recollect the comfort of sitting by a fire warming ourselves when it's cold or remember the brightness and heat of a sunny summer's day. When there is no fire and warmth around us, the world can seem a gloomy place. We might feel cold and distant and life can appear dreary, bleak and cheerless.

The sun is a source of warmth and light for the earth. Flowers, plants and trees need heat and sunshine in order to grow and flourish. The summer, which is the season associated with Fire, is when flowers are in full bloom. The same is true for us. In order for us to bloom with vitality and radiance, we need the qualities of a strong Fire Element.

People who are constitutional Fire types will have both capabilities and negative traits associated with their Element. For many Fire types the extremes of joy and misery may be familiar. The saying 'laugh and the world laughs with you; cry and you cry alone' might have been written by a Fire type.

THE BACKGROUND TO FIRE IN CHINESE MEDICINE

Introduction

The Fire Element consists of the concept of Fire and its key associations. These are:

Organs	Heart, Heart Protector, Small Intestine, Triple Burner
Spirit	Shen — the mental-spiritual aspect of the Fire Element
Colour	Red
Sound	Laughing
Emotion	Joy
Odour	Scorched

These associations are discussed in more detail later in the section. Understanding them will help us to recognize Fire types and understand the connections between the Organ and the Fire type's behaviour patterns which are described later.

The Organs of the Fire Element

The main Organ associated with Fire is the Heart. We will also refer to the:

♦ Heart Protector, which is the protector or guardian of the Heart and in a Western sense corresponds to the pericardium
♦ Small Intestine, which the Chinese described as the 'Separator of the pure from the impure' and
♦ Triple Burner which is more a function than an Organ in Western sense.

Remember what we said in the Wood type chapter. The Chinese described Organs metaphorically, as in the term 'Heart Protector', and also functionally.

The Heart and the Heart Protector

Chinese Medicine describes the Heart as the 'Supreme Controller'. The Heart was compared to an emperor who the Chinese regarded as half-god and half-human. It was via the emperor that the Chinese felt they had a connection with the Heavens and the world of spirits. This term 'Supreme Controller' is very apt as one of the jobs of the Heart is to make sure the other Organs, such as the Liver or Lung or Kidney, function harmoniously.

In real life, if the emperor lost control of the nation it became chaotic. As a person, if our Heart becomes imbalanced, we may feel 'out of control', extremely anxious, jumpy or panicky inside. If on the other hand the Heart or emperor is well balanced, we will feel peaceful and settled inside.

The function of the Heart is so important that it has the Heart Protector to support it.[1] The Heart Protector is rather like the guardian of a gate which leads directly to the Heart. A guardian who is healthy will open the gate to let in any positive, loving and beneficial experiences and will also close it to keep out any negative, toxic and harmful ones. The appropriate opening and shutting of this gate stops the Heart from being injured, but allows it to take in warm and nourishing experiences.

The Mental-Spiritual aspect of the Heart

The importance of the Heart is partly explained by the 'Shen' which is the mental-spiritual aspect of the Heart. In the same way that the Wood Element is associated with the Hun, which is our 'eternal soul' or life plan, the Fire Element has the 'Shen' which is sometimes translated 'mind' and sometimes 'spirit'. The Shen is said to have four functions:

♦ To make us fully conscious — in the sense of being physically and emotionally self aware
♦ To help us think clearly — to be able to think a problem through with a clear objective and to speak coherently
♦ To have a good memory — this is in the short-term sense of not being absent minded and knowing where our keys are or remembering the name of the person we just met
♦ To sleep well — especially being able to drop off to sleep quickly and sleep deeply

The Chinese said that the Shen resides in the Heart. Any imbalance of the Heart means that the functions of the Shen will be impaired.

The Small Intestines and Triple Burner

The Small Intestine is nicknamed 'the sorter'. Its physical job is to receive food from the Stomach and separate out the 'pure' or desirable nutrients from the 'impure' ones. It also has an important mental or spiritual job. Everyday we take an enormous amount of 'food' for our mind — through personal and social contacts, television, newspapers, magazines, films, the internet and many other sources. What should we keep; what should we throw out?

This 'sorting' is the job of the Small Intestine and it can easily become overloaded by all the organizing it has to do. A weakened Small Intestine may quickly find a job too much, and we end up feeling fuzzy-headed, muddled and unable to think clearly. For example, a person who is important to us makes an ambiguous and possibly hurtful remark. We are confused at the time and go away thinking about it. Over time we find we cannot process it; we cannot separate the pure from the impure. Like a piece of undigested food, it remains in our psyche's digestive tract.

The Triple Burner is a 'function'. Chinese medicine describes three 'burners' or processing areas which lie in the chest, the solar plexus area and the lower abdomen. They are called the upper, middle and lower burners respectively. One of the jobs of this 'function' is to keep the organs that lie in these areas in balance and harmony. So, in that sense, the Triple Burner shares the function of the Heart.

THESE SYMPTOMS MAY ARISE WHEN THE HEART AND PERICARDIUM ARE WEAK OR OBSTRUCTED

Some of these symptoms are more physical and some more mental or of the spirit. Chinese medicine being 'energetic' does not make this an important distinction.

Anxiety, palpitations, panic attacks, insomnia, poor concentration, poor memory, pale lips and a propensity to startle easily. Breathlessness, daytime sweating, listlessness, a pale face or cold limbs. Mania, excessive restlessness and extreme confusion. Stuffiness or pain in the heart region.

Observable Signs of a Fire Type

Signs which indicate that a person is a Fire type are the following:

♦ A pale colour on the face — usually at the side and under the eyes, but sometimes over the whole face; also a frequent flushing up of the whole face from pale to red and back.

♦ A scorched odour — resembling burnt toast, ironing or clothes from the tumble dryer.

♦ A laughing sound in the voice — as if the person is about to giggle; alternatively no laughing and a monotonous, miserable tone.

♦ An under- or overjoyous emotional state which will be referred to in a later section.

Postures, Gestures and Facial Expression

Over time the Fire type's chronic emotional state can become moulded into their postures and gestures or 'etched' onto their faces.

Many Fire types have a slightly under-developed chest area, especially if the Heart or Heart Protector is the main Fire Organ affected (see Figure 7).

Sometimes the chest looks slightly caved in or the top half of the body may be less strong or skinnier than the other parts of the body.

We may also notice that the posture of joy is much more upwards and expansive than the posture of sadness which can often be slumped. Sometimes a Fire type can have very changeable movements which range between being expansive and upwards and more withdrawn and slumped. Similarly, the face alternates between lighting up with joy and dropping into sadness (see Figure 8).

Facial expression can also be indicative of a Fire type. Many Fire types smile and laugh a lot. A smile will not, however, truly express joy unless the eyes are also involved. Sometimes, when a Fire type smiles, the eyes can really sparkle with joy. Other times, the real joy is missing and the eyes don't shine. In some Fire types, whatever the face does, the eyes seem chronically sad and the corners of the mouth have become fixed in a miserable, downward droop.

Fire types sometimes find it difficult to look another person in the eyes. If the Heart is too open, they feel vulnerable making contact.

THE EMOTIONAL CAPACITY OF THE FIRE ELEMENT

The Fire Element has a capacity which has an important effect on our emotional life:

♦ The ability to give and receive warmth and love with varying degrees of emotional closeness.

A strong Fire Element gives us the ability to open up to become intimate with others or to close down to be distant. Coupled with this is the ability to detect just how much to open up or close down. Knowing 'when and by how much' is of course partly due to experience. If we have a well-balanced Fire Element we will easily make these relevant perceptions.

A Fire Type and Relationships

We all need to form relationships of different kinds. Oliver James says that:

> There is a vast body of evidence proving a fact of which few of us can be unaware: that we have a powerful drive to form intimate relationships and that if these relationships turn sour or end it puts us at risk of a variety of problems.[2]

Relationships vary enormously. Some relationships are ones we consciously choose, for example a 'life partner', in which case we usually have an 'intimate' relationship. Others are friendships either with people of the same or a different sex but which involve no physical intimacy. Some relationships are ones we do not consciously choose, although they may be close. For instance, our relatives are people we relate to because they are 'family' and colleagues because we see them on a daily basis.

Role-based relationships, for example, with the bank manager, the plumber, the doctor or dentist, are naturally more formal and not intimate. 'Formal' does not mean unfriendly, but the Heart is concerned with when and how much to open up.

Becoming Close to Others

The Fire Element is particularly important when developing a close relationship. When we first meet people we can have a range of different reactions. Sometimes we immediately 'warm' to another person and intuitively feel that we could get close. Sometimes we instinctively shy away. Our Heart is discerning.

Whatever our initial impressions the actual *process* of forming a relationship takes time. A relationship often starts off quite formally. There was a time when it took people some time to get on to 'first-name terms'. Nowadays many of these formalities have been dropped but we still need to progress from a stage of relative formality to less formality. If appropriate this can go on to more closeness as we get to know another person.

Opening up our Heart Protectors

As this process moves forward our Fire Element and our Heart and Heart Protector slowly allow us to open up. They enable us to develop a relationship of trust and caring at the appropriate level. If we find that a person cannot be trusted, we can close down to a slightly more formal level. The depth and rate at which we draw close to others varies from individual to individual. It can only happen if our Fire is functioning in a balanced way.

Although our Elemental imbalance is constitutional in origin, our early experiences will affect the way they manifest. Next we will look at what happens when the Fire type becomes imbalanced.

EMOTIONS WE EXPERIENCE WHEN THE ABILITY IS IMPAIRED

If our Fire is imbalanced, then our ability to give and receive warmth becomes impaired. We may easily feel shut off from others or become too open. Sometimes we may open up or close down to others at inappropriate times. As a result we may become:

♦ Miserable and vulnerable
♦ Fluctuating in our emotions
♦ Muddled and unable to sort things out

We will talk about each of these in turn.

Feeling Miserable and Vulnerable

Being too open can lead a Fire type to feel extremely vulnerable and sensitive to others. They can easily feel hurt or wounded at any signs of rejection. This may range from feeling slightly upset at one extreme to feeling utter devastation and betrayal at the other. Here Sally describes the feelings that have been with her all her life:

I've had a sort of feeling of rejection and betrayal all through my life and there is definitely a wound whenever I get upset. There is a wound and also an unmet need and there is also a negative belief about myself that ties it all together. When things get bad I try to find the unmet need and do something about it.

In terms of our progression through life, the root of vulnerability often begins in childhood with what is perceived as rejection or abandonment. Beliefs get formed about one's vulnerability or need for 'love' and these in turn support further experiences of hurt and disappointment.

The more the Fire Element is imbalanced, the more the gates controlled by the Heart Protector become stuck open or closed. When they are stuck open, the smallest offence — being let down by a friend, ignored momentarily by family or left out by those at work — causes hurt. When they are kept closed, then intimacy is not achievable and real warmth and love evade the Fire type. Clare describes the problem which gets created:

I protect myself from betrayal by not opening up to people so I can't get hurt. If people don't give anything back it's really hurtful, then I get cold inside. I just hate it when people don't respond.

When our Fire Element becomes really imbalanced we can completely lose any spark of emotional warmth — in this case the expression 'cold hearted' may be very apt. As Joan said:

When I become really sad I become cold and go quiet — it's not like purposefully sulking, it's just that I am so hurt that I become kind of cold and dead.

Our Fire 'going out' can also cause us to feel extremely sad and joyless as Pat described:

One state I often get into, when I'm really low, is not being able to laugh at all. Someone might crack a joke and I want to be able to laugh but I can't as I'm so miserable.

THE IMPORTANCE OF OUR EMOTIONAL TIES

Studies carried out on more than 37,000 people show that social isolation — the sense that we have no one with whom to share our private feelings or have close contacts — can increase our mortality rate significantly. A report in 1987 in *Science* showed that mortality from isolation is a greater health risk than smoking!

Studies also show that there is a corresponding drop in the mortality rate of those people who have strong emotional ties. Of patients who had a bone marrow transplant 54 per cent who had strong emotional support survived after two years as opposed to only 20 per cent of those with little support.[3]

Fluctuating Emotions

Fire types often have changeable emotions. They may oscillate between joy and sadness — the two main emotions associated with the Fire element.

At one extreme when a Fire type is feeling joyful, they fill everyone they meet with warmth and excitement. They can have what seems to be an almost in-built ability to 'sparkle' especially when other people are enjoying life with them. At their best they can be life's natural optimists who can enthuse and see positivity in the worst situations. Gail told us:

On a good day I can enthuse others — I'm infectious in the enthusiasm — it's a little like lighting other peoples' fire with my own. With my light I can brighten up other peoples' shade.

At the other extreme Fire types may feel really gloomy and miserable and unfortunately this too can be catching. Gail continued:

The downside is that I can feel really low at other times and then I drag others down and put their fire out.

The fluctuations often relate directly to other people. A Fire type might wake up feeling miserable. Later they may meet someone who is nice to them or who gives them a compliment and they feel much better. Later their mood may go up or down again depending on the quality of the contact they have with others. For some Fire types when they are feeling 'up' it can be so good that they do not care that they will fall down flat later on. Jane expressed this well:

It is like being on a cloud, you just float along high and you know you might fall off but you don't mind because it's so good being on top of the cloud.

Others can find their changeability disconcerting as Pat explained:

My feelings are inconsistent. I can be crying into my pillow one minute then someone will phone and I'll say, 'Oh I'm fine', and I *am* actually fine. When I noticed this I thought, 'How weird that I can't trust my feelings', but it's just that my feelings keep changing rather than I can't trust them.

When the Small Intestine is the most imbalanced Organ, the Fire type may experience problems to do with discrimination.

Feeling Muddled

If the Small Intestine Organ is imbalanced then this may result in difficulties in 'sorting out'. Earlier in the chapter we described how the Small Intestine allows us mentally to separate 'pure' from 'impure'. When this organ is out of balance the Fire type may feel blocked up in the head, mentally fuzzy or have difficulty thinking clearly. They will be unable to prioritize, feel uncertain about what they think and unsure as to what is important. Charles, who has a 'sorting' problem, told us:

I tend to have difficulty differentiating between what's important and what's not. The result is that I tend to do everything. For example, I write articles for journals and I'll put in every single reference as I can't discriminate between what to use and what to leave out. When it comes to women I get bowled over by beautiful women really quickly and can't sort out between the 'good' the 'bad' and the 'ugly' at all! And that leads to problems.

Rachel also said:

I often feel confused and have difficulty seeing things clearly. It's like having dirty windows which I can't see through. Then when I feel better it's like the windows have been cleaned.

THE BENEFITS OF HAPPINESS AND LAUGHTER

Happiness and laughter can help us to ward off infections. A study asked 72 people over a 12-week period to fill in questionnaires about how their day had been. Those people who had laughed a lot or who had experienced a good day had a higher level of an antibody called 'immunoglobulin A' in their systems. This antibody was correspondingly lower when people had had a bad day, leaving them more open to colds and other infections.[4]

Recognizing the Emotion of a Fire Type in Everyday Life

We might recognize Fire types by the way they express, or do not express, their joy. A common observation is that the Fire type's joy is stimulated by someone external, but the joy generated seems to have no life of its own. Rather than rising to a peak and settling smoothly, it drops and disappears quickly, often to be replaced by a look of sadness. Alternatively, in extreme cases, whatever we do, it seems impossible to generate even the slightest smile in them — like blowing on the embers of a fire which has already gone out.

Many Fire types may also seem to crave compliments and attention. These feed their Fire and make them feel worthwhile and happy. They may also feel warmed up if they are hugged by someone they care for. Julie told us:

I love getting hugs. I just need cuddles — and I'm *not* talking about sex — just needing cuddles. I suppose it's very childlike.

Another very positive possibility is that we may find our own joy being lifted time and time again by the Fire type. The Fire type cares about happiness and will often go to great lengths to lift the spirits of those around them.

BIG ISSUES AND UNANSWERED QUESTIONS FOR THE FIRE TYPE

For any type, when typical negative experiences recur, certain issues become more important than others. The Big Issues for the Fire type are:

♦ Craving love and warmth
♦ Emotional stability

♦ Happiness
♦ Closeness

To say that these are the Big Issues is to say that in any situation, particularly ones of stress, the Fire type will automatically be concerned with giving and receiving warmth and love, finding emotional security within themselves, finding happiness and joy and finding closeness with others. Depending on the strategies the Fire type has chosen, some of these will be more important than others.

Another way of expressing the internal experience of someone whose Fire is constitutionally impaired is that they begin, to varying degrees, to carry certain unanswered questions such as:

♦ Am I lovable?
♦ How can I find a good relationship?
♦ What can I do to be noticed?
♦ How can I feel happy?
♦ How can I become emotionally stable?

For the non-Fire type, there are answers to these questions. For the Fire type, these questions keep recurring and to varying degrees do not get answered. The difficulty in finding answers can lead a Fire type to develop various life patterns or strategies.

HOW WOULD YOU KNOW YOUR FRIEND IS A FIRE TYPE?

She or he might:

♦ Look pale at the side of the eyes
♦ Have a face which flushes red and back at frequent intervals
♦ Laugh a lot or not at all, or go from one to the other
♦ Love it when you are genuinely warm and friendly
♦ Both enjoy closeness and sometimes be nervous of it
♦ Sometimes seem up and sometimes down
♦ Be easily hurt by a harsh comment

RESPONSES TO THE BIG ISSUES

The ways of coping which we will discuss next are a response to the Big Issues and Unanswered Questions. Given that these issues are important and the questions keep recurring, these are the kinds of lifestyles or behaviours which a Fire type might adopt to deal with their issues.

Not every Fire type will use all of these strategies and there may be other variations which we have not observed. It is also possible for other types to behave in similar ways. In this case the behaviours might be less pronounced or have a different set of questions behind them.

The responses are:

♦ Being cheerful
♦ Clowning and performing
♦ Opening up inappropriately
♦ Becoming isolated
♦ Closely relating

Being Cheerful

The question 'Am I lovable?' can lead to Fire types trying to please everybody around them. Usually this is such an unconscious part of their nature that they won't even realize they are doing it. Fire types are often described as 'the nice guy', 'friendly lass' or as the 'cheerful person' who brightens everyone up. Underneath, however, the Fire type can feel very uncertain about their own likability. Here Clare points out:

In party situations there's a constant undercurrent of insecurity and anxiousness and I think it's masked by a sort of happy and jolly outward expression. I want everything to be nice and everybody to like me.

Because many Fire types feel vulnerable and easily slighted they can become sensitive about hurting other people. Instead of standing back and seeing things in perspective they might immediately blame themselves if someone else is upset. Ben told us:

Sometimes I'm ultra-sensitive. I pick up if other people make the slightest pauses. It may be they're tired and I think, 'Have I done anything to upset them?' It's like you kill yourself over this and they're probably just a bit tired.

Happiness is a big issue for Fire types. Deep down they hope that if others become happy then they too will find happiness and be contented. If the 'vibes' around them are bad they can feel very uncomfortable. Sorting things out could cause a row. For a Fire type this is often preferable to remaining in a negative situation. The *best* scenario, however, is pleasing others and keeping the vibes good. This strategy does not always work of course. A Fire type may remain positive, cheerful and nice when others are feeling ratty or depressed. In this case they may end up defeating the object and causing another row. A colleague commented:

I think if you are in the right mood or need cheering up it can be really nice to be around a Fire type, but if you are not in the right mood it's quite annoying.

Being nice does not always energize a Fire type either. It can be a strain which leads to them feeling drained. Jennifer said:

It's the thing that is underlying everything. I want people to like me — even if it's really dumb because I don't really like them. Sometimes it can be quite exhausting.

If Fire types do not feel lovable or if they want to be noticed, another strategy may be to become a clown.

Clowning and Performing

We've all seen Pierrot, the clown with the teardrop gently flowing down his face. He is happy on the surface but sad underneath. If we are unhappy and depressed we can cheer up other people by becoming a clown. At the same time we can also cheer ourselves up. Here both Mike and Sue describe making people laugh. Mike told us:

When I first went to school no one seemed to like me and I felt very insecure and lonely. I found that if I was naughty I would get a laugh and people started to be friendlier, so I became the class clown.

Sue said:

I would pretend I was stupid when I wasn't — if I did silly things like be cheeky in class, or pretend I didn't know anything I thought people would like me more.

Many comedians are Fire types — Eric Morecambe, Benny Hill, Tommy Cooper, Les Dawson, Tony Hancock and Frankie Howard to name a few. Interestingly, they have all been popular comedians — and most of them have died from heart problems. Eric Morecambe and Tommy Cooper had heart attacks while they were on stage! Benny Hill loved to make people laugh and was literally 'heartbroken' when he was told that his show was not going to get another series — he died only a short time later. Making people laugh and keeping people entertained can help some Fire types to feel that they are worthwhile and lovable.

Others who love to act or are in show business may also be Fire types. They may revel in the adoration, attention and love they get from their fans and often come most alive when they are on stage. Underneath, they may lack confidence and be very unsure of themselves. They know they're lovable only when their audience gives them admiration and attention.

Some Fire types find other ways of performing or clowning even though they are not on stage. Some people's stage is the rostrum they lecture from, the pulpit they preach from or the office where they play the fool to their colleagues. They may not get overt applause but any praise or appreciation from their 'audience' helps them to feel that they are lovable, worthwhile people.

Opening up Inappropriately

Some Fire types so desire to relate to everybody that they lose their discrimination. They may no longer sense when it is applicable to open up to people and when it would be more appropriate not to. Janice told us:

My partner is really open and often he doesn't know who he is with. Like he'll have a conversation about the finances of his company with the cleaner or something. It seems inappropriate but they're highly entertained — he's probably just sorting out his own thoughts and having an open conversation with himself.

Appropriate openness is in part a subjective judgement, but experience and wisdom suggest that whatever our feelings, we proceed with some care when developing an intimate relationship. Fire types sometimes jump right into a close relationship, failing to go through the 'normal' stages or formalities. The consequences are the test. A succession of aborted relationships does not usually produce satisfaction or develop self-esteem.

Fire types could be the ones who tell a roomful of strangers about their personal life and difficult relationships. Alternatively, they might feel personally rejected by the bank manager who won't give them a loan. They may overlook their lack of financial plan or the fact that finances are tight. The bank manager has made a business decision; the Fire type experiences a personal slight.

Another consequence of extreme openness may be regularly falling in love with someone who is obviously unavailable or someone inappropriate, like the DJ at a party. Crushes occur in our teens even though we may not act on them. In our thirties and upwards, if falling in love happens every two weeks, it should be considered inappropriate. Sometimes this inappropriate behaviour of a Fire type can be viewed as charming by the person on the receiving end.

Others may find it less appealing and the Fire type may be rebuffed. For some Fire types this may be a hard lesson to learn. They may persistently and repetitively get hurt until they learn to distinguish between a fleeting passion (which might be the basis for a one-night stand) and the possibility of a relationship (which requires slower development). The Fire type who has frequently been rebuffed may shut themselves off from the world and become isolated.

Indeed, this characteristic is close to the ability to contact and influence others almost instantaneously. President Clinton is known for being able to make deep contact quickly and influence voters. His ability to have an open heart contributes to this skill, whatever else it does for him.

Becoming Isolated

Problems with our Fire Element can lead us to have difficulty relating to the people around us. Fire types may hide away from the world and become introverted and unsociable. They can be afraid to develop friendships because they anticipate rejection and hurt. The closer they become to other people, the greater the possibility of betrayal.

Many Fire types seem outwardly friendly but are closed off internally. They may be incapable of forming deep friendships and only allow others to know them on a superficial level. The result is no deep relationships, but the payoff is that they do not get hurt, betrayed or rebuffed. They may fear the hurt which could come from getting close to others and so decide not to have close relationships at all. Unfortunately, as Oliver James points out, we could be putting ourselves at risk of feeling sad and depressed, developing compulsions, e.g. an eating disorder or violence.[5] Paula told us:

> One thing I can't make happen is relationships so now I spend a lot of time alone. Maybe it's easier to be by myself than to keep getting rejected. But I do get very lonely at times and I comfort eat a lot.

Many Fire types yo-yo between wanting to be on their own and wanting to be noticed by other people — resulting in a major conflict. As Jenny told us:

> I find I have a contradiction between the desire to be seen and not seen. It is quite a powerful one. I find I have a wardrobe of brightly-coloured clothes and I have crazy haircuts and then I say 'Don't look at me!'

At the other extreme to becoming isolated are those Fire types who place their highest priority on the closeness they feel with others.

Closely Relating

Gerry is someone who likes to feel bonded and close to others:

> My work is about connecting with people — it's like food for me. I like a community around me; it's very important. I want to be nice and for us all to love each other — my life is very much to do with me relating to others.

Some Fire types do not feel whole unless they have constant one-to-one deep connections with other people. This may steer them towards a variety of situations. It may lead them to be constantly networking and making contact with others. At the extreme this may seem to be promiscuous as they become close and intimate with many different people. In this case the connection of the moment takes priority and other commitments are forgotten. Later on this could create severe repercussions in committed relationships which become hard to sustain because of jealous and upset partners.

Others are searching for the 'perfect' relationship. They may be disappointed when they realize the partner of their dreams is also human with many faults. Yet others want a relationship so badly that they immediately open up their hearts to a new friend or potential partner before finding out if the person can be trusted with their heart. The result of this, as we noted in the previous section, can be that the Fire type ends up getting hurt and feeling that they can never sustain relationships.

The need to relate can also lead some Fire types to become exceptional in work with people. They may become therapists, counsellors, members of the clergy or involved in other one-to-one work. This satisfies their need for deep connections with others.

Some Fire types may find it difficult when other types do not have the same needs for closeness as them. They may end up feeling pushed away or rejected by others because they seem too needy. In this situation they may find other ways of fulfilling this need. Here Sam describes how she has turned to another kind of faithful friend who never betrays her:

I'm quite needy and that's why I get such a lot from animals. People find it hard to be constantly giving whereas dogs can. They are so enthusiastic and they love you and when you come home they kiss you. Mine do anyway. You are not going to expect your loved one to jump up and kiss you all over — so I've found a way of feeding my needs that does not encroach on humans.

These are the key ways that Fire types bring love and warmth into their lives. Most Fire types will have a combination of different strategies. They may be hiding their feelings away one day, only to become too open the next.

VIRTUES AND VICES OF A FIRE TYPE

Depending on the health of the Fire type, the ways of coping produce both virtues and vices. Some of the virtues are:

♦ A capacity to bring sparkle and joy into other people's lives
♦ An ability to relate closely to others
♦ A capacity to be optimistic in the most difficult circumstances
♦ Being able to lead by enthusing others
♦ A commitment to finding inner peace and contentment.

Some of the vices are:
♦ Feeling easily hurt, sensitive and vulnerable
♦ Feeling miserable and unable to laugh
♦ Superficiality and an inability to make deep intimate contact
♦ Volatility and fluctuating emotions
♦ Relating to others out of context and inappropriately.

A FAMOUS FIRE TYPE — MARILYN MONROE[6]

So famous is she, that when people hear the word 'Marilyn', an image of Marilyn Monroe usually comes to mind. She was vulnerable and sweet and at the same time sexy and seductive. It was her many Fire type characteristics which led her to become a screen goddess. She had the combination of the ability to be cheerful and also of 'clowning'. In the film *Some Like it Hot* she showed a genuine flair for comedy. Like other Fire types she was also inclined 'to open up to others inappropriately' and would often get involved in unsatisfactory relationships. At the other extreme she could become isolated when times were bad.

Her early life exacerbated all the insecurities and feelings of rejection that made her a Fire type. She often felt, and indeed was, abandoned by those who were caring for her. Throughout her childhood she spent a lot of time with foster parents and in orphanages. This made her feel extremely vulnerable and easily rejected. She never quite believed that she was lovable or beautiful but it was also this vulnerability which somehow contributed to her fame as an actress.

She had a difficult childhood. In spite of this, as we said above, she was also the typical 'cheerful person' and was described as being a 'winsome child with ash-blonde hair and an engaging smile and bright clear eyes'. At the same time as being cheerful she could also become quite bleak at times and was known to daydream and fantasize in order to make up for the lack of love in her life.

Along with other Fire types she was also a natural performer and was encouraged by an old friend of her mother's to set her sights on becoming a movie star. The friend, Grace, taught her to pose and look good and to take care of her appearance. Marilyn learnt from an early age how to play to a crowd. Like many other Fire types she sparkled when given attention. At the age of thirteen she became aware of her ability to attract and fascinate men. As she changed from child to voluptuous woman, she loved to walk to school waving to all the men who hooted at her as they passed in their cars.

When being photographed she also knew how to play to the cameras. Being in front of a camera brought her Fire Element to life. It was said that, 'When she saw a camera she instantly lit up. Then when the shot was over she fell back to her not very interesting pose'.

Many Fire types pay a lot of attention to their relationships. Many also have difficulties with them. Marilyn was no exception. She first got married when she was sixteen and went on to marry three times and to have many lovers, including President John F Kennedy. Her first husband described her as 'sensitive and insecure' and said that she could easily feel hurt. He also said, 'She thought I was mad at her if I didn't kiss her goodbye every time I left the house.' Like many other Fire types she endlessly needed to know she was loved by him but she also feared his rejection. She could also be oversensitive — her Heart Protector did not protect her from the hurts and knocks of life.

Typically of someone so vulnerable, she chose unsuitable partners. She gradually became bored by her first husband and left him. Her second marriage only lasted for nine months and her third to Arthur Miller also ended in divorce. People have speculated that by repeating the unhappiness of her past she thought she might reverse the effects of her unhappy upbringing. Sadly, if this was what she set out to achieve, she did not succeed.

Marilyn became increasingly unstable as her life progressed and later, before her death, was dependent on alcohol and pills. Suspended by her studio for her absences and lateness she finally died of an overdose of sleeping tablets in 1962. The world mourned her death. In her life she worked to resolve her sadness, but did not succeed. She was a beautiful, but sad, star who became an icon for the 20th century.

GOLDEN RULES FOR FIRE TYPES

Remember, close contact with others nourishes you.

♦ Take care of your level of openness: discriminate between different people and different contexts.

♦ Know what you want from others and know what they want from you.

♦ Know what context you are relating in and therefore how others will understand you.

♦ Ask yourself, 'What will happen when I discover I am lovable?'

Notes

1   It is reasonable to ask why the Chinese spoke about both the Heart and the Heart Protector separately, rather than putting them together. Traditional Chinese medicine teaches that there are channels or pathways of energy running through the body. Each pathway is associated with an Organ. One of these is associated with the Heart and the other with the Heart Protector and for this reason they are given different although related functions.

2   James, Oliver, 1997: *Britain on the Couch*; page 133.

3   'Social Relationships and Health', James House et al. Published in *Science*, July 29, 1988.

4   'Secretory IgA antibody is associated with daily mood', A Stone, D Cox, H Valdimarsdottir, L Jandorf and J Neale. Published in the *Journal of Personality and Social Psychology*, volume 52, May 1987.

5   James, Oliver, 1997: *Britain on the Couch*; page 133. James refers to research indicating that broken relationships often lead to depression, violence and compulsions, especially eating disorders.

6   Spoto, Donald, 1994: *Marilyn Monroe, The Biography*; and various authors, 1998: *Biographical Dictionary of Women*.

Chapter 5

EXERCISES FOR FIRE TYPES

INTRODUCTION

The exercises in this section are aimed at enabling Fire types to find a better emotional balance. Some useful goals for the Fire type are:

- ♦ To appreciate the different contexts of their relationships
- ♦ To know the process of developing a relationship in addition to recognizing passion
- ♦ To believe that they are lovable and to love themselves
- ♦ To stabilize their emotions
- ♦ To feel happy and peaceful.

USING THE EXERCISES

We suggest that you read an exercise through before you start it. All of the exercises are laid out in a similar style. Following the *introduction*, we tell you approximately *how long* it will take to complete. Obviously some of you will take more time and others less. The exercises are then divided into stages. They start with:

- ♦ the *purpose* of the exercise and then
- ♦ the *process* or the steps of the exercise.

The theme of each step is in bold so that you have a summary. At the end of some exercises we have a section called *'matters arising'*. Here we discuss issues which could come up while you do the exercise.

THE EXERCISES FOR FIRE TYPES

+ Discovering you are lovable
+ Building relationships with the people in your life
+ Entering an intimate relationship
+ In a relationship — ask for what you want!
+ Resolving our feelings of shame
+ Taking pleasure from the world
+ Releasing sad feelings
+ The inner smile
+ A Qigong exercise for the Heart.

EXERCISE 1 — DISCOVERING YOU ARE LOVABLE

Introduction

Jenny had a history of not feeling fulfilled or loved in relationships. She was unsure about whether she had picked the right partners or whether she would ever be happy in a relationship with anyone. Her current relationship had lasted two years, but she was having a familiar and difficult time around not feeling loved.

The first time Jenny did this exercise, she found a lot of feelings coming up which she said were centred around her heart and which she expressed through tears. She was not sure what they were about. As suggested, she repeated the exercise several times. As she did this, the feelings lessened in intensity and in between doing the exercises she spontaneously remembered incidents when she had doubted whether her parents really loved her. In the end, she completed steps 4, 5 and 6 of the exercise. Later she told us that the difficulty she was having in her relationship passed and she says she is feeling positive about it continuing.

Time needed: 10–20 minutes.

Purpose

Fire types sometimes do not believe they are lovable and this exercise helps you to experience yourself as lovable. It addresses the confusion which arises if you doubt that you are lovable and wonder if another person really loves you. Believing in your own lovability comes first. Whether a specific person loves you or not is then easier to determine.

Process

1 **Find a person for whom you feel love — the kind of love you would like to receive yourself.** The love can be in your personal life, but can also be for relatives, friends or children.

2 **Find out 'how you think' about this person.** To do this, find an image of the person and check the following areas:

   ♦ Where do you see the person — straight in front of you, to the left or to the right?
   ♦ Do you see the person at eye level, above or below?
   ♦ Is the picture moving or still, black and white or in colour, is the person face/half-body or full body?
   ♦ How far away is the picture?
   ♦ Do you hear the person's voice and if so from where?

Make some notes about how you represent this person. For instance, the picture may be straight in front of you, at eye level, have slight movement in it, be in full colour and be about three feet away. The person in the picture may be speaking. This is the way you think of someone for whom you feel love.

3 **Now, put an image of yourself in the 'lovable' place.** However you see yourself, make the qualities of your image the same as those of the image in step 2. By doing this you are seeing yourself in the same way as you see someone you feel love for.

4 **Let yourself know you are lovable.** If you feel comfortable looking at yourself in the 'lovable' place, then simply say, 'I know you are lovable. Which means I am lovable.' Notice how you feel saying that. Then say, 'I love myself'.

   If feelings do arise, just hold the image of yourself and the feelings. Allow them both to be there. If you cannot hold the image of yourself, then just allow the feelings to be there. The feelings may be ones of hurt. If so, think of these feelings of hurt and sadness releasing and clearing your heart. You may find it helpful to say: 'As the sadness comes out, you are becoming lovable. I know I am lovable.'

   If this stage has generated a lot of feeling, then you may wish to leave the exercise for a while. When you return, put yourself in the 'lovable' place again and allow any further feelings to arise. You could do this several times and each time you will get closer to knowing that you are lovable — 100 per cent.

5 **Know why you are lovable.** If stage 3 was smooth, see yourself in the lovable place and ask: 'What does she/he have, that makes him/her lovable?'

Collect the answers and then put yourself in the lovable place again and say for each answer to the previous question: 'She is lovable because ...', inserting the answers after 'because'.

6 **Notice what you have received from this exercise and how to carry on.** You may have responded in differing ways. Often in stage 3, specific incidents from the past can come up. These may be ones which, if they were stuck inside you, could keep you believing that you are not lovable. Repeated releasing and the understanding which comes from the exercise can be helpful. The only thing that can make you unlovable is believing so.

EXERCISE 2 — BUILDING RELATIONSHIPS WITH THE PEOPLE IN YOUR LIFE[1]

Introduction

One day Harry said to his friend Dean how important people are. Dean, who felt that Harry had neglected him on occasions, laughed and asked, 'How come you don't care more for people like me then?' Harry told his friend Dean not be stupid, but later in the day he began to wonder about Dean's remark. After talking to several other people, an acquaintance of Harry's (he had a lot) suggested this exercise. Six months later Harry actually thanked Dean for saying what he had. Dean obviously did not quite remember, but he touched Harry on the arm and said, 'Hey, you're my buddy. I like you. Remember that!' Harry felt good inside.

Time needed: 15–25 minutes.

Purpose

The purpose of this exercise is to consider the people in your life and how you can build close and productive relationships with them. If people are important to you, they are worth some time and thought. Throughout the exercise write your answers down.

Process

1 **List the important people in your life, however many there are.** These are people who are relevant to your happiness and welfare. They can be partners, friends, work colleagues, neighbours or any other significant people.

You may mention groups. If you are a teacher, you could pick out individual students and/or just say 'students'. From the list, select an important person as a subject of this exercise. When you appreciate the results of this exercise, you might choose to repeat the exercise using other people from your list.

2 **Take one important person in your life and describe what kind of relationship you want with them.** To do this, ask the following questions:

a) What **goals** do I have? For example, you might say:

♦ I want a *special* friend so I can feel close to someone outside my family

♦ I want a squash or football buddy

♦ I want someone to go to the pub with and just chat

♦ I want a girlfriend who I can feel close enough to, to talk about our relationship

♦ I want a supportive business relationship

b) what qualities do you want present in this relationship? list things like:

♦ friendliness

♦ trust

♦ interest in football, butterflies, sports, etc.

♦ closeness, empathy and sharing of personal information

c) What is the **context of this relationship?** With what frequency, when and in what places will this relationship take place? Answers can be varied, e.g. daytime at the office; in the evening, a couple times a week, at the sports club or in the pub; or almost anywhere, anytime.

d) **How will you know** that you are getting what you want? What will you be seeing, hearing or feeling that tells you? Be as specific and realistic as you can.

3 **Find some goals that you both share.** If you share a goal, this automatically builds the relationship. These can be such things as:

♦ keeping your wardrobes up to date

♦ getting better at aikido

♦ keeping informed about changes at head office

♦ informing the neighbourhood about 'green' issues

♦ learning how to use your computers

4 **What can you do to make this relationship happen?** Because the relationship involves two people, you cannot automatically make it happen. It also depends on the other person's response to you. So start with two changes in your point of view.

First, put yourself in the other person's position. (See Wood type exercise number 2, The Other's Point of View). In this position, ask yourself what would make you want to be in such a relationship. Make any notes you need.

Secondly, put yourself in the Objective Point of View. (See Wood type exercise number 3, The Objective Point of View). When looking at yourself and the other person, ask 'What does X (your name) need to do to foster this relationship?' Again make notes. List whatever actions you need to take to promote or nurture this relationship.

5 **Aim to generate positive feelings in the other person.** Recall the ways that others have made you feel good, e.g. by:
   ♦ talking about what you like to talk about
   ♦ complimenting you
   ♦ doing small favours
   ♦ remembering your birthday or an upcoming interview

   Make a list of things you can do to generate positive feelings in the other person and then carry them out.

EXERCISE 3 — ENTERING AN INTIMATE RELATIONSHIP

Introduction

Sally was a single mother, with a daughter of seven, having divorced five years before. Since the divorce she had had many short relationships. The pattern seemed to be that Sally would fall instantly and passionately in love, but the relationship which started never seemed to last. She desperately wanted a lasting and committed relationship.

Sally worked through this exercise with her acupuncture practitioner over five weeks. She was not sure at first about the value of the exercise. But one day she came in and said, 'Thank you, I met the most wonderful man two nights ago and I thought to myself "I love him, but can I have a relationship with him? And am I going to work on that?"' It was clear that the exercise was beginning to pay off.

Time needed: 20–30 minutes.

Purpose

This exercise is for those of you who are not in a relationship (or are maybe just beginning one). If you have a tendency to fall in love quickly and passionately (how else?) and later get abandoned, hurt and dispirited, then this exercise may give you another approach.

Process

1 **Think about how a house gets built or how a baby grows into an adult.** This is a process which has stages which are important at different times. The moment of 'love at first sight' and a moment ten years later with three children and financial problems are different. We require different skills to deal with them.

2 **Make your own list of the stages of a relationship,** based on your thoughts about how a house gets built, how a baby grows into an adult and your own experience. It is important for you to think about what is right for you. This is not how we say it might be or how it has been for you in the past. Here are some ideas but there is no standard process. Some of the stages people suggest are:
   ◆ first contact
   ◆ attraction
   ◆ first agreed 'date'
   ◆ getting to know about the person and their history
   ◆ some touching, deeper eye contact, expression of pleasure in the other's company
   ◆ more regular dating
   ◆ some statements of commitment
   ◆ sexual intimacy
   ◆ discussion of a long-term relationship
   We stress that there is no standard pattern for building a relationship and any stages you think of must respect your ethics, culture and your experience of the world.

3 **Set some criteria or standards for each stage.** We suggest you do this by specifying your stages — five are probably enough — and then for each stage find three important criteria under the following headings:

The information and understanding the other person needs to have about you. *'What I want you to know about me is ...'*
The information and understanding you want to have about them. *'What I want to know about you is ...'*
This might include:

♦ personal likes and dislikes
♦ occupation, interests and hobbies
♦ any other close relationships
♦ previous history (especially of relationships)
♦ family
♦ relation to important people in the present and past, for example, parents, brothers and sisters, previous partners
♦ beliefs about self
♦ what is perceived as important in a relationship
♦ The boundary rules for you or any agreements you would expect to make. *'What I want understood or agreed at this stage is ...'*
This might include:
♦ how you behave to each other in public or private
♦ whether to acknowledge to others the connection you have
♦ how you relate to others
♦ when to let each other know where you are or have been
♦ whether to allow each other into your private worlds
♦ how you show respect for each other

Use a sheet of paper and write down the first stage as a heading. Underneath put down everything to do with your criteria or standards.

It is hard to specify the whole list because it all depends on what is important to you in a relationship. There will be many things which you expect of your potential partner's behaviour and attitudes. Think of what these might be and write them down.

You may need to work through this several times to find the information, understanding, boundaries and rules which are right for you for each stage. You may be helped in the overall process by talking to friends, especially ones who you believe have good relationships.

WHAT I WANT FROM A RELATIONSHIP

Stage 1. First contact
What I want you to know about me
What I want to know about you
What I want agreed or understood

Stage 2. First date
What I want you to know about me
What I want to know about you
What I want agreed or understood

Stage 3. Getting to know you
What I want you to know about me
What I want to know about you
What I want agreed or understood

Stage 4. More regular dating
What I want you to know about me
What I want to know about you
What I want agreed or understood

Stage 5. Sexual intimacy
What I want you to know about me
What I want to know about you
What I want agreed or understood

4   **Use the standards you have set.** Having done this exercise once, look at what you have written on a regular basis and compare it with your behaviour. If you are beginning a new relationship, ask, 'Which stage am I at and what would I like to be happening at this stage?'

Matters Arising

Any discussions you have with other people are aimed at shaping your own views, rather than taking on other people's ideas. Writing these down and questioning their importance is going to change your later behaviour. Some Fire types skip stages of relationships. If you have skipped stages, without getting the relevant knowledge, understanding or agreements from a partner, you may begin to appreciate that this has caused you emotional pain. It may also have stopped you from getting what your really want — stability and warmth.

EXERCISE 4 — IN A RELATIONSHIP, ASK FOR WHAT YOU WANT!

Introduction

Brenda and Lesley worked in the same office and always had lunch together. They talked a lot about their respective partners and Lesley had a constant complaint: Will said he loved her, and maybe he did, but somehow he did not quite do the right things — he just did not understand what Lesley really wanted. Brenda took Lesley through the following exercise. Lesley found it easy to describe what she wanted, but felt uncomfortable about asking Will to express himself differently. To her surprise, when she asked Will to behave differently in a specific way, he just said, 'Sure, I can do that.' And he did. Lesley was taken aback, but she got the point and began regularly to ask for what she wanted. Not surprisingly, Will began to do the same. Eighteen months later, they both think it has had a very positive effect on their relationship.

Time needed: 15–20 minutes — longer if the exercise becomes a habit.

Purpose

One of the main sources of problems in a relationship — any sort of relationship — is that we tend to assume that others want what we want. We fail to recognize our differences. For example, one person may regard someone making them a cup of tea and giving them thoughtful presents as a sign of love and appreciation. Another person may want to *hear* that they are loved and *hear* that someone understands how they are feeling. Someone else may regard all these as insignificant and has other 'signs of love'.

We are assuming for this exercise that your relationship started with mutual attraction or benefit, has had its periods of satisfaction and there is still good will between you. We are also assuming that rather than describing and explaining what is wrong, it is better to work co-operatively for a win/win solution. This means that both partners get what they want.

If your partner is not willing to work with you on this exercise, then work on your own in the way described below. Working with a good heart will soon clarify in your own mind whether the two of you can recreate something worthwhile.

Process

1) **Recognize what not to do to make things worse**. It is easy, when you don't get what you want, to complain, explain, criticize or blame.

- ♦ **Complaining** is expressing dissatisfaction with what your partner has or has not done. It does not usually bring closeness, understanding or satisfying new behaviour.
- ♦ **Explaining** is finding reasons for why things are not working out. It includes such things as 'you are always too busy' or 'your mother trained you badly'. However interesting explanations are, they do not usually lead to solutions.
- ♦ **Criticizing** is finding fault and varies according to the harshness with which it is done. Harsh criticism is never solution oriented.
- ♦ **Blaming** is saying that what is going wrong is your fault, not mine. Again, finding who is to blame does not lead to solutions.

One of the first things to do is to withdraw your energy from complaining, explaining, criticizing or blaming. Otherwise it is as if there is a sign-post which is pointing in one direction and you are walking in another.

2 **Now, ask yourself 'what makes me feel loved?'** (If 'loved' is not the right word for this relationship, then substitute 'appreciated', 'I have a friend', or whatever is appropriate. Write these down. It may help you to do this if you remember times when the relationship was really good.

Make your answers specific and use the following guidelines. First of all, two 'don'ts':

- ♦ Don't say that you want the other person to *feel* something
- ♦ Don't say what you do *not* want the person to do.

Now, four 'do's':

- ♦ Ask for behaviour
- ♦ Describe the behaviour specifically as if you had seen and heard it on TV
- ♦ Focus on *actions* such as 'buy me flowers' or 'ask me how I am and be prepared to listen for five minutes', or on *voice tones*: 'talk to me in the way you talk to so and so', or on *voice volume*: 'talk gently and quietly', or on facial expressions 'I love the way you looked at me when Joseph was first born', or on *gestures and ways of touching*: 'I like the way you put your arm around my waist and squeeze me', or on *specific words and phrases*: 'I love it when you say I am special.'
- ♦ Be prepared to write down the words or phrases you like, demonstrate the gestures, voice tone or volume and write down a list of actions.

The goal of this is twofold. One is to know what behaviour would satisfy you. The other is to be able to describe this behaviour in a way that the other person can understand.

You may go through this stage several times. When you ask yourself, 'What do I want?' you will probably discover things and learn better how to communicate them. Most people who have done this find the ability to say what they want develops and improves with practice over time.

3 **Consider how and when to communicate.** First, remember that other people may have an entirely different set of needs. They may like things *said* to them and you may like things *done* for you. They may appreciate being touched in a certain way and you may appreciate being touched in an entirely different way. Appreciate that if they are different, they may not easily take in what you want. They may not easily believe you. They may not feel they can even do what you want. So consider that you are talking to someone from a different planet — if the thought has not already occurred to you.

Secondly, choose a good moment to communicate. Ideally when the other person has time and is in a good mood. *Ask* for the time and whether it is OK now. If not, ask when will be a good time. Explain what this is about. In general, give the communication its best chance.

4 **Monitor your progress, don't expect miracles and reward progress.** It will be natural to notice progress or otherwise. If the other person is doing something that they have not naturally done before, then accept even small changes with gratitude. To do this, acknowledge and reward the person. You can be specific and say something like: 'I really appreciated it when you (describe the behaviour specifically). Thank you. I liked that.' Realize that at that moment you are increasing your likelihood of getting what you really want!

5 **If possible, set up a regular time to discuss mutual satisfaction.** If you start to get what you want, then you could arrange to meet regularly. Your agenda might be: What do we want from each other? What do we appreciate about each other? You may even find that your life changes and what you want may start to change too.

EXERCISE 5 — RESOLVING OUR FEELINGS OF SHAME

Introduction

Annie's practitioner noticed that she'd never say what *she* wanted. She would answer a question about what she wanted in a situation either by saying what she thought other people involved wanted or by saying she really didn't know. One day her practitioner asked, 'what would happen if you were definite about what you wanted and simply told everyone else?' Annie looked panicky and said she could never be like that.

In the discussion that followed, she said that on many occasions she felt ashamed of herself and even embarrassed about mentioning her shame. When asked if she would like to explore her shame without having to expose it and she said, 'Yes'. After going through the following exercise once, she said that for the first time in ages, she felt good about herself and was it possible to use it again? Over several weeks, she said her shame, which had been around as long as she could remember, was getting much, much easier. Finally she said that she now knew how to deal with whatever came up — all by herself.

Time needed: 20–30 minutes.

Purpose

This exercise is the most effective way we know of helping people to overcome their feelings of shame. When we are ashamed we feel that we are 'bad' in some way because we have ignored other people's standards.

Until their shame is resolved, people often fear that they will be rejected or abandoned if they reveal it. Because of this fear of rejection we have put this in the exercises for Fire types. Of course any type could find this exercise useful. Please note that even if someone else helps you to do this exercise, you don't have to tell them the reason why you feel ashamed.

Process

1 **Think of what makes you ashamed.** This can either be something you're *ashamed of* or it could be more that you may feel *ashamed of yourself generally*.

Become aware of whatever image the shame brings up in your mind. It may take a while for you to find an image. Don't worry. Take your time. Make sure you see or sense yourself in the picture as well as any other people involved.

2 **Notice the qualities of this image including:**
   ♦ Its colour, size and distance from you
   ♦ Its location — to the left or right or directly in front of you
   ♦ Is it moving or still?
   ♦ Are there any sounds or words in the image, if so where are they coming from?
   ♦ Notice yourself and the other(s) in the image and *especially your size in relation to their size.*

Often people who are ashamed see themselves as smaller than those who have disapproved of them. The disapproving people are often in a fixed position and staring at them in a belittling or reproachful manner.

3 **Now think of another time, this time where you ignored someone else's standards but you didn't feel ashamed about it.** This could be a time you disobeyed someone but it didn't matter, or you were 'cheeky' or feeling slightly rebellious. We will call this the 'positive image'.

When you have found a positive image, notice the qualities this brings up in your mind. *Make sure that you and the other(s) in this image are the same size.* Notice as well the size, colour, distance, location, movement and sounds as before. You might find you have some kind of protective shield around you in this image. If you do not have a protective shield, feel free to give yourself one.

4 **Now transform the 'shame' image into the positive image.**
   ♦ Change any distortions to yourself in the 'shame' image. People who feel ashamed often distort the image they have of themselves.
   ♦ Make yourself the same size as anyone else in the picture.
   ♦ Change the position of your picture until it is in the same place as the positive image.
   ♦ Transform its colour, size, distance, movement and/or sounds so that they are similar.
   ♦ Give yourself a shield to protect yourself. This is like giving yourself a 'Heart Protector' (see page 64 Chapter 4).

5 **Look again at the situation that made you feel ashamed.** Notice if it creates the same feelings of shame. If it does, go back to your two images and check that you have fully changed the shame image into the positive image. If you haven't completely changed your shame image, do anything necessary to create a better match.

If you find you no longer feel ashamed, well done! There are only two more short steps for you to do.

6 **Examine your standards.** Remember that the reason we feel ashamed is *that we have ignored standards that others have told us we should have and which are not our own.* Ask yourself some questions about the situation that made you ashamed such as:

♦ What was the standard I ignored that caused me to feel ashamed?
♦ Was this my standard or someone else's standard?
♦ Do I want this standard?
♦ If I don't want this standard, what alternative standard can replace it?
♦ Is this new standard one which I would want others in my life to use?

7 **Imagine yourself acting according to your new standards in the future.** See yourself in a variety of situations. Go through this exercise again to deal with any other shameful experiences. You can use the same 'Positive image'.

Matters Arising

Shame is sometimes called the 'hidden emotion'. That's because when we feel ashamed of something we are likely to hide it and feel unable to talk about it to anyone else. It can then be hard to resolve our feelings. Shame is probably one of the most debilitating emotions we experience and we often end up feeling ashamed about being ashamed.[2]

EXERCISE 6 — TAKING PLEASURE FROM THE WORLD

Introduction

Godfrey is a Fire type and he often complained that he went up and down emotionally. He also frequently focused on want was wrong and the negative aspects of his life. We suggested that he tried the following exercise to train his attention on positive things and create stability. After two months of keeping the morning and evening journal, Godfrey was asked about going up and down. He smiled.

Time needed: A few minutes every day

Purpose

At any moment in time we usually have a choice as to what we notice or think about. This exercise encourages us to develop a 'half-full' mentality, focusing on what gives us satisfying and pleasant feelings. Everyone can benefit from doing this simple exercise. It is especially useful for Fire types, however, as it will enable them to feel steady from day to day and become conscious of what makes them happy on a deep level.

Process

Keep a journal of the things you enjoy and appreciate on a daily basis. It may help to answer these questions.

In the morning on waking ask yourself:

+ What do I appreciate in my life at present?
+ What am I enjoying about my life at present?

In the evening you can ask yourself:

+ What have I learned from today?
+ What positive things have happened today?
+ What have I given out today?

EXERCISE 7 — RELEASING SAD FEELINGS

Introduction

Jenny was mentioned in the introduction to Exercise 1. In that exercise she learned something about releasing feelings of sadness which were interfering with her capacity to feel lovable. She also learned more from this exercise as to how to keep her heart and chest area open and clear.

Purpose

There are times when Fire types feel unhappy and that their feelings of sadness have become caught inside them. It may be hard to cry and the Fire type may then go around feeling miserable until the feelings are released. This is not so much an exercise but more a practical suggestion as to how to let go of pent up feelings.

Process

If you are feeling miserable and the feeling is caught up around your Heart, a good weep may be needed. **To release the feelings you may take up one of these suggestions:**

+ Go to see the saddest film you can find.
+ Rent a number of weepy videos and watch them one after the other.
+ Read a moving book.
+ Watch pictures on the news, or anywhere else, of those who are much worse off than yourself.
+ Read some sad poetry.
+ Go and see a good friend who will listen to you. Tell her or him all the things which are making you miserable. Make sure that the friend agrees to listen to you and does not give advice or try to 'fix it' for you.
+ Do the 'Focusing' exercise in chapter 3, on page 43. This will give you more insight into what is causing you to feel sad. You might then be able to let go of the feelings.
+ Go outside and stamp your feet on the ground. You might be surprised about how much this simple movement can change your feelings or help you to release them.

The aim of these suggestions is to help you to get your feelings out of your system. Sitting and moping about your problems usually only makes them worse, so it is best to try doing something positive. Once you have had a good weep or got the feelings out of your system you may once more feel able to cope with the world.

Clearing emotions can be an important release, but they will recur unless you also deal with the underlying causes. You may now wish to do some of the other exercises for Fire types in order to create equilibrium at a deeper level.

EXERCISE 8 — THE INNER SMILE

Purpose

This is a well-known Chinese exercise which only takes a few minutes to do. It is very simple but can be profound in its effect. It is recommended for everyone, but is especially beneficial if you are a Fire type. It will perk you up if you are feeling flat or low. The exercise will also relax and rejuvenate you and will make any difficulties easier to cope with. You can do this exercise at any time — sitting in the office, in a stressful meeting or when studying for exams. It can also be used to prepare you for Qigong exercises.

Time needed: a few minutes.

Process

1 **Imagine seeing, feeling or hearing something that makes you smile.** This might be recalling something pleasant from the past, seeing someone you feel good about, remembering a time you felt happy or cared for, recollecting a time when someone gave you a compliment or remembering someone making a joke.

2 **Allow yourself to smile internally** — it doesn't have to be visible — only felt by you. If you feel so flat that nothing makes you smile then act as if something has made you smile.

3 **Allow the smile to shine out of your eyes, then let the smile travel downwards into all of your internal organs.** Notice the feeling of relaxation generated by the internal smile. Allow the smile to travel down to your lower abdomen just below the naval.

4 **Continue what you have been doing but keep the feeling generated by the internal smile.** You might find that others will also respond to the good feelings activated by your internal smile. This in turn will make you feel happier.

QIGONG EXERCISE FOR THE HEART

Purpose

This exercise stretches the chest and also settles and relaxes the Heart and Pericardium.[3]

Time needed: About 5 minutes a day.

Process

1 **Stand with your feet shoulder width apart and the inside edges of your feet parallel.** Keep your knees slightly bent. From your hips, bounce gently up and down, about an inch or two. Feel how your weight travels down from your hips to your feet which are solid on the floor. Tuck your tailbone in so that your lower back is straight. Draw your chin in slightly so that your spine stretches upward. Relax your chest and let the front of your abdomen drop.

2 **Now place your hands, palms facing inwards, on your lower abdomen.**

3 **Bring the palms up to the chest at the same time as taking a breath in.**

4 **Extend your arms horizontally out to your sides,** at the same time as exhaling. Imagine your breath flowing out through the tips of your fingers, especially the little finger which is the energy pathway of the Heart.

5 **Bring your hands back to your lower abdomen and repeat the exercise.** Continue doing this exercise for at least five minutes. See Figure 5.

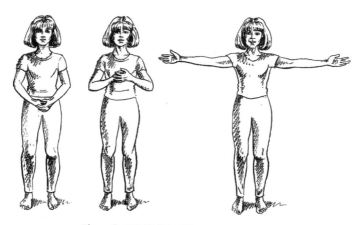

Figure 5: QIGONG EXERCISE FOR THE HEART

Notes

1 This exercise has been adapted from Andreas, Steve and Faulkner, Charles, 1996: *NLP, The New Technology of Achievement*; pages 141–7.

2 For more about Exercise 6 on resolving our feelings of shame see Andreas, Connirae and Andreas, Steve, 1989: *Heart of the Mind*; Real People Press, Moab, Utah, Chapter 14, pages 140–54. The shame exercise has been derived from this source.

3 This is adapted from an exercise in Sandra Hill, 1997: *Reclaiming the Wisdom of the Body*; Constable, Great Britain.

Chapter 6

THE EARTH TYPE - NOURISHING OURSELVES

MARTINE IS AN EARTH TYPE

Martine is an Earth type. Her face has a yellow hue and she has a slightly sing-song voice tone. She is also very good at caring for people and others often turn to her when they need help. Here she talks to us about being an Earth type.

There are positive and negative sides to being an Earth person. One of the positive things is my ability to be caring and mothering. Before I knew about Chinese Medicine I thought other people sometimes disapproved of the way I mothered my children and that I was over-concerned for them and supported them too much. When I heard about Earth types I thought, 'Yes, this is me and this is all right!' As far as I'm concerned my children are for ever and not for five minutes. They're a part of my life. Although they've grown up we're still attached because they're a part of me.

I also love to feed people and look after them. When people come to visit I adore cooking for them and making them feel at home. I also love nature, being with the earth and gardening. In fact anything to do with being with nature is really good for me.

Martine also admitted that there are negative sides:

One of the negative sides is being over-sympathetic and looking after people too much. I can get into terrible trouble if someone's telling me a tale of woe.

I'll jump in and say things like, 'How can I help, do you need any money, what can I do?' I try and help *too* much.

I also find I'm sometimes very sympathetic to other people but I can get disappointed if others aren't sympathetic back to me. I have to take a deep breath and remember that not everyone's like me. I've also heard it said that Earth types are quite needy — of course I get needy at times. I used not to like it, but now I can say, 'Well this is me and it's OK.'

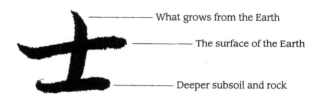

Figure 6: THE CHINESE CHARACTER FOR EARTH

THE EARTH ELEMENT IN NATURE

The Chinese character for Earth is Tu (see above). The top line of this character represents the surface soil of the Earth and the line below it the subsoil or rock deep underground. The vertical line characterizes all of the things produced by the Earth.[1]

So, based on this simple character, how do the Chinese understand Earth? What does the Earth provide for those of us living on its surface.

The Earth supplies both nourishment and stability. Much of the food we eat is grown and harvested from the Earth. If the soil is of good quality we will receive nutritious food. If the soil becomes polluted or deficient, so is the food grown from it. 'Mother' Earth then fails to provide us with high quality food and we are no longer nourished properly.

The Earth also provides us with stability so that we have a solid base beneath our feet. In rare circumstances, we lose this stability. Brenda was involved in the earthquake which took place in California in the early 1990s. Here she tells us of her experience:

I went into kind of awe — something so much bigger than me was taking place — my whole body was being shaken, almost as if the Earth was rocking me. For the next few months whenever there were aftershocks I could feel it in my stomach like it was physically being shaken up.

We receive food and nourishment on many different levels. We need physical food as well as mental and spiritual food. Our human mothers or carers are our first providers. They feed us with milk when we are young and also with comfort and support when we need it. This nurturing helps to create good quality 'Earth' within us.

If we grow up well-nourished and secure physically, mentally and spiritually we will be able to experience ourselves as being centred and stable. We can be nourished by those around us and in turn nourish them.

In this chapter we will be looking more deeply into how the Earth Element provides us with nourishment and stability. We will also find out what happens when it becomes imbalanced.

THE BACKGROUND TO EARTH IN CHINESE MEDICINE

Introduction

The Earth Element consists of Earth as it is represented in the character and all of the Earth associations. The important associations are:

Organs Stomach and Spleen
Spirit   Yi — the mental-spiritual aspect of the Earth Element
Colour   Yellow
Sound   Singing
Emotion Worry and sympathy
Odour   Fragrant

Familiarity with these associations will help us to recognize Earth types and understand the connections between the Organ functions and mental processes described later.

The Organs of the Earth Element

You will remember from previous chapters that the Chinese give a metaphorical description of the Organ and then a more specific description in terms of the energy or 'Qi' of the body and mind. Both the Stomach and Spleen have functions to do with assimilation and nourishment and, roughly speaking, equate to our digestive systems. They are the two main Organs governing the creation of our energy. Both have functions which go beyond the purely physical, however, and it is important to remember that they are also associated with the Yi (pronounced yee) which is the mental and spiritual aspect of Earth.[2]

The Stomach

The Stomach is the organ in charge of 'rotting and ripening' our food and drink. Its function is like a cement mixer, processing the cement and sand. When making concrete, correct ingredients are important. But the mixer itself must do a proper mixing job. Either poor ingredients or poor 'rotting and ripening' will result in a weaker material. In the one case we have a structurally unsound building, in the other a weakened body and mind.

We also rot and ripen mentally, when digesting and assimilating information. Sometimes our mental 'mixers' work well. At other times, we turn things over and over, obsessing and worrying with no useful output. We end up in a state of mind that some Earth types describe later, where our heads are fuzzy and we feel unclear.

The Spleen

The Spleen is called the 'Transformer and Transporter' of all the food, drink and other substances in the body. The 'transformer' refers to the Spleen's role in converting food and drink into new cells and replenished energy. The 'transporter' refers to the Spleen's role in carrying the nourishment transformed from our food to every part of the mind and body. If the Spleen is weak, then our digestion slows down and food and fluid starts to accumulate. These excess fluids can make us feel heavy in our body, limbs or head and muzzy-headed mentally.

A poor Spleen function will also manifest in bloating after we eat and can change our appetite. We may go off our food or have an 'abnormal' appetite. This may mean we only wish to eat poor quality food, such as fast foods or sweets and crisps, rather than food which is nutritious. When the Spleen malfunctions we will not be nourished adequately. We can start to get weak in our limbs and feel extremely lethargic.

The Spleen houses our 'Yi', the Earth's mental and spiritual aspect.

The Mental-Spiritual Aspect of Earth

Yi is translated as 'thought' or 'intention'. The Yi gives us our capacity to think, study, concentrate and memorize. If the Earth Element is imbalanced and the Yi is weak, then this can result in learning difficulties, fuzzy thinking, poor concentration and an inability to put our thoughts into action.

In Chinese medical treatment, strengthening the Spleen can be used to improve mental functioning. As practitioners, we have found this to be true. The effect goes both ways. A poorly functioning Spleen results in poor mental function, but excessive mental functioning, for instance, studying for exams, can stress and weaken the Spleen.

Many Chinese Qigong exercises involve our Yi and aim to strengthen it at the same time. For example, one exercise involves pushing outwards with our hands. To do this more effectively we can imagine a mountain in the distance and that the energy of our hands can touch and push it. Indeed, Qigong exercises almost always use and strengthen our Yi — and thereby affect the functioning of our Earth Element.

If our Yi is functioning well, we will be enabled to 'reap a harvest' from our lives. This means we are able to fulfil our dreams and get our needs met. If we are unable to do this we may end up feeling chronically 'starved' or undernourished physically, mentally and spiritually.

THESE SYMPTOMS MAY ARISE WHEN THE STOMACH AND SPLEEN ARE WEAK OR OBSTRUCTED

Some of these symptoms are more physical and some more mental or of the spirit. Chinese medicine being 'energetic' did not make this an important distinction.

Poor or excessive appetite; an appetite only for poor quality food; discomfort in the stomach area, nausea, loose stools, a bloated abdomen (especially after eating). Weak limbs, prolapsed organs, tiredness especially after eating. Worry and obsessive thoughts. Muzzy head, poor concentration, a desire to lie down, heaviness and a stuffy feeling in the chest or abdomen.

Observable signs of an Earth type

In addition to the symptoms mentioned above, there are some keys signs of an Earth type. These are:

♦ A yellow, earthy colour to the side and under the eyes and on the side of the cheeks.
♦ A singing sound in the voice where there are frequent ups and downs (some languages, e.g. Welsh, tend to have a 'sing song' tone so take this into consideration).
♦ A body odour for which the English translation is 'fragrant' while the actual odour is a cloying one which sticks in the nose.
♦ The person's emotional expression, which we will deal with in a later section.

Posture, Gestures and Facial Expression

An Earth type may be physically weak around the area of the stomach and spleen and tend to place a hand over the area as if giving it comfort or support. They may look slightly collapsed in that area. Carol notices this is accentuated when she is tired:

When I'm tired or ill I tend to slump in my middle. I don't normally notice that I feel weak in that area — only when I'm feeling under par. Whenever I sit down with a hot drink I hold the cup against my stomach — it's almost as if I'm unconsciously trying to warm myself up there, it feels very comforting.

Some Earth types have large, slightly flabby bodies, the result of poor 'transformation and transportation'. This is most obvious in the thighs (cellulite) or the lower and middle abdomen which may be associated with feeling of fullness after eating.

Our legs connect us to the earth and some, though not all, Earth types have poor energy in their legs. Their legs may be thin and underdeveloped or more bloated and flabby. In either case, they are unable to make full contact with the energy arising from the Earth. There is more about this in Chapter 7, Exercises for Earth types.

Earth types are often caring and sympathetic and the associated feelings can often be noticed on their face and in their gestures. The facial expression is very soft. The eyes have often been described as gentle, like a 'puppy dogs' and the eyebrows are slightly raised which may cause small lines to appear on the forehead. There is often an accompanying tilt to the head when empathizing with others.

Worry, which is also associated with the Earth Element, mainly shows itself on the forehead which creases into a frown. The eye may be defocused showing that we are lost in our own internal world as we chew over our problems.

THE EMOTIONAL CAPACITY OF THE EARTH ELEMENT

The Earth Element gives us an ability which we can describe in the following way:

♦ The capacity to take in support and nourishment as well as to support and nourish others appropriately.

Taking in Support and Nourishment

When we are young our mother or a mother-figure feeds us, holds us and provides for us in many ways. If we fall and hurt ourselves she comforts us and administers to our wounds. If we are anxious, she calms us and if we are hungry, she feeds us. This nurturing is part of our developing a strong centre, a good sense of ourselves and the ability to literally 'stand on our own two feet'. If we have well-balanced Earth energy it is easy for us to respond to this nurturing.

As we grow and mature, what counts as support and nourishment changes. We evolve from being suckled by our mother to feeding ourselves. Feeding ourselves can be taking in nourishment on many different levels. It can include asking for support when we need it and feeling cared for when a friend acknowledges that we are having a tough day.

Giving Support and Nourishment

The capacity of the Earth Element is to give as well as to receive. We are social animals and, with respect to support and nourishment, achieving a balance between giving and receiving is crucial. If we have developed a strong centre and can nurture ourselves, in turn we will support those around us. We will also be empathetic and caring when the need arises.

A strong Earth Element does not mean, however, that we will give uncondi-tional support to others at all times and as soon as they ask for it. Good farmers know that after growing crops, the earth needs to lie fallow. The earth replenishes itself, something the farmer cannot do for it. Overuse and over-fertilization of the soil will deplete it and it will no longer produce high quality food. If our Earth Element is balanced we will be able to distinguish between times when it is appropriate to look after the needs of others and times when we need to nourish and care for ourselves.

EMOTIONS WE EXPERIENCE WHEN THE ABILITY IS IMPAIRED

When our Earth is imbalanced we are less able to give and receive nourishment. This can affect us in a variety of ways and we tend to experience:

♦ Cravings for support, sympathy and understanding
♦ Struggling to assimilate
♦ Worry and over-thinking

Cravings for Support, Sympathy and Understanding

A young child falls and hurts itself. Its first reaction is to run to its mother or main carer for comfort. Even if there is no noticeable injury the mother rubs the affected area better. The care relieves the child's pain and it can go and play again, secure in the knowledge that mother is there whenever more support is needed.

If the mother pushes the child away or ignores its pain for a lengthy period of time, then the child will feel permanently in need of the care and support it never received.

The Earth type's imbalance is constitutional. Their ability to receive support and nourishment is less robust and they are likely, therefore, to need more. As a result, they are more inclined to end up feeling they have not been given enough — and, in the end, they may develop an unfulfilled need for support, nourishment and sympathy.

Some Earth types come to believe that their own needs are insignificant compared to other people's. Jan describes this:

I know I am over-sympathetic and this makes it hard for me to focus on myself. I feel very needy, but it's a struggle for me to think of my own needs as being as important as everybody else's. Somehow that makes my own needs seem even larger.

Others develop an outlook which interferes with the normal process of nourishment and stops them from getting what they want. Moira describes some of the beliefs which clearly prevent her receiving appropriate support and nourishment:

> No one can ever really give me what I need. If I really revealed my needs to people they'd run a mile because they're unsatisfiable. I hate feeling I need anything and if I showed my needs, I know I'd be in someone else's power and be too vulnerable.

THE POWER OF EMOTIONAL SUPPORT

A study was carried out at Stanford University in 1989 on women with advanced breast cancer. The findings were stunning. Women who attended meetings where they could talk to others with similar problems, survived for twice as long as those who didn't. The only difference between two groups of patients in the study was that the group who met regularly could unburden themselves of their worries and knew they were with others who understood and were willing to listen to them.[3]

Struggling to Assimilate

As we stated earlier, our Yi is the mental and spiritual aspect of the Spleen. Roughly translated, Yi is our intention or our ability to think clearly. When the Earth is imbalanced, our Stomach cannot 'rot and ripen' and our Spleen cannot 'transform and transport'. In consequence our thoughts become unclear. Laura told us:

> It comes and goes, but there are times when I need to think and I'll feel my mind just scrambling. My head feels like a confused jumble and it's a real struggle.

Moira also describes the inside of her head as an 'impenetrable thicket':

> Sometimes I can't think clearly or can't think through something. It's like an impenetrable thicket. I can't think my way through it. It's too much effort to

think through. Then it's best to wait until I feel clearer. On a good day I can plough through a lot in one go and it's really enjoyable.

Some Earth types report that they do not have the energy to follow things through. There is a process whereby we think something through, form an intention and then carry it out. But the Earth type can falter in this process, and have good ideas but not put them into practice. The effect is not to reap a harvest. Another Earth type described it:

> I am lying there knackered and somebody has a great idea and I think, 'yeah, let's do that', but then I just feel I can't be bothered — something doesn't connect. Like my thinking and my body do not connect.

EMPATHY IN OUR EARLY LIFE

Daniell Stern, a psychiatrist at Cornell University, studied how mothers connected to their children. Some mothers consistently avoided empathizing when their child expressed a need for a cuddle or was in tears. This in turn took a tremendous toll on the child's ability to express emotions. The infant avoided expressing or perhaps even feeling those emotions themselves. Stern does say, however, that there is hope for them to be repaired as relationships throughout our life continually reshape us.[4]

Worry and Over-Thinking

One translation of the emotion associated with Earth is 'over-thinking'. Although we might not call 'over-thinking' an emotion, it does describe an emotionally driven process of chewing something over and over — like a cement mixer which is unable to mix the sand and cement. Here Moira describes what happens to her:

> I have to go over and over and over things. I am sure it must be terribly irritating. If I've got anything on my mind I have to talk about it and talk about it and talk about it until it is processed. That can sometimes take quite a long time.

Patrick relates his over-thinking to feeling insecure:

I think everything through more than other people and I can think it, sort it, file it then sort it again — I'm better these days I'm not so insecure, but I still do it.

Worry, which is another description of over-thinking, is often felt in the Earth type's stomach area. As Anne told us:

I can sometimes feel very worried; it's like a big unease in my solar plexus area. I can't do anything about it until the situation has resolved. I always have this feeling when my daughter's away.

Assessing the Earth Type's Sympathy

In everyday life, how would we recognize the emotional expression of an Earth type? Worry and sympathy are closely connected. It is normal for us to want sympathy when we have a worry or difficulty. We may talk to others about our problems and they empathize and let us know they understand. The difference for Earth types is that their worry or need for sympathy will be more excessive than other people's.

Many Earth types freely admit to being worriers. If you ask, 'Do you worry?', they often say, 'Oh yes, all the time.' When you ask 'What do you worry about?', they might say, maybe smiling 'Anything, it doesn't matter.'

Earth types might also talk more about their problems than others. Asking them, 'How are you?' could result in a twenty-minute discussion. They might also need larger quantities of concern from other people about their problems. Other Earth types may be unable to take in the concern shown to them. For example, when someone has complained and you give some genuine understanding or sympathy, do they digest it or 'take it in'? (Remember the associated Organs!)

Another response is that, in spite of asking for, or in any case appearing to need, support, they might reject your sympathy out of hand, for example, by saying that they are fine and there is no real problem. This response will seem odd as you will have judged that they really are in line for just a little bit of sympathy or support.

One patient we knew had a very debilitating illness. He refused all understanding and practical help. Although he could not do up his shoelaces, he would not let others help him. He even hated someone saying, 'Take care'. The phrase offended him — he would not have people giving care or showing understanding to him. This was an extreme case.

BIG ISSUES AND UNANSWERED QUESTIONS FOR THE EARTH TYPE

For any type, when typical negative experiences recur, certain issues become more important than others. The Big Issues for the Earth type are:

♦ Feeling supported
♦ Getting nourished
♦ Centredness
♦ Mental clarity
♦ Being understood

To say that these are Big Issues is to say that in any situation, particularly ones of stress, the Earth type will almost automatically be concerned with feeling supported and nourished by others, feeling grounded or centred, feeling clear mentally and being understood by those around them. Depending on the strategies the Earth type has chosen, some of these will be more important than others.

Another way of expressing the internal experience of someone whose Earth is constitutionally impaired is that they begin, to varying degrees, to carry certain unanswered questions such as:

♦ How can I get centred?
♦ How can I get the support I need?
♦ Who will nourish me?
♦ How can I get what I want from the world?

For the non-Earth type, there are answers to these questions. For the Earth type, these questions keep recurring, and to varying degrees do not get answered. The difficulty in finding answers to these questions can lead an Earth type to develop various life-patterns or strategies.

HOW WOULD YOU KNOW YOUR FRIEND IS AN EARTH TYPE?

He or she might:

♦ Look yellow at the side of the eyes
♦ Have a voice tone which goes up and down
♦ Give you all kinds of support and help
♦ Over-smother you with care and concern
♦ When things are even slightly bad, complain a lot as if seeking sympathy
♦ Look either under- or over-nourished
♦ Be heavier in the lower part of their body
♦ Feel tired and sometimes say they can't think

RESPONSES TO THE BIG ISSUES

The ways of coping which we will discuss next are a response to the Big Issues and Unanswered Questions. Given that these issues are important and that the questions keep recurring, these are the kinds of lifestyles or behaviours which an Earth type might adopt to deal with their issues.

Not every Earth type will use all of these ways of coping and there may be other variations which we haven't observed. It is also possible for other types to behave in similar ways. In this case the behaviours might be less pronounced or have a different set of questions behind them.

The responses are:

♦ Mothering and caring
♦ Not asking but expecting
♦ Expressing needs a lot
♦ Searching for a centre
♦ Homemaking

Mothering and Caring

Two of the big issues for Earth types are support and nourishment. What better activities to engage in than mothering and caring? We mean these terms in the widest sense. Thus an actual mother may engage in mothering and caring, but so also might a social worker, pastor, teacher, prison officer or a community worker. Neil, an Earth type, describes the impulse:

I'm always mothering and being thoughtful. Like an acquaintance is coming in from San Francisco tomorrow so I'll meet him — I think of things like that. Today I heard that one of my friends' dads is in hospital and I thought, 'I'll ring him.' People said 'You can't do that — his dad's dying,' but I thought, 'If it was me I'd like it, so I'll do it.' I am always thinking of things to do for others.

Another way the Earth type can fulfil a need to care for others may be as a parent. Many Earth types have conflicts around the mother figure and feel they didn't get supported and nurtured when they were young. They can, however, adore homemaking, families and children and find great fulfilment in raising them. Sarah said:

I love mothering and I loved being pregnant and having babies and giving birth and I love being around little kids. I even helped set up a birth centre in my home town. I felt really desolate for a while when child rearing was over.

Some, but not all, Earth types can be found in the caring professions working as doctors, nurses, therapists, counsellors or complementary therapists. There are also many other jobs where caring is involved. They may, for instance, serve as a shop assistant, answer the phone as a receptionist, work in the service industries or do voluntary work — the impulse to care can be directed into many areas of their lives.

An Earth type can be in the wrong job, however. We know of one Earth type who worked for a bank and audited the business of several branches. Auditing requires financial objectivity, but she was so concerned about the feelings of the manager and staff of the bank being audited, that she was in serious conflict.

If the impulse to care for others goes to an extreme, it can become more of a need for the Earth type, than for the person they are caring for. The Earth type may then be trying to support others who are not asking for help — or requiring it. This kind of mothering can lead to smothering as Inga pointed out:

I think one thing that makes me difficult to live with is that I can actually be over-nurturing, over-bearing and over-mothering. And some people don't actually like that. They feel smothered and they want to get out from underneath.

Some Earth types who are 'carers' may work on doggedly. They may care for the unfortunate, the 'victims' and needy of society that others have ignored or given up on. This can result in them looking after people inappropriately and not always being careful about who it is. Carol told us:

> I used to take on people who would do me no good. I'd think, 'I must do something for this person', even though they might not be a nice person. I'd even invite tramps home for supper. I'd be feeling sorry for people inappropriately.

The 'caring' Earth type who goes to extremes faces burn-out. Caring too much for others and not enough for oneself is a danger. We have encountered many 'carers' who, in spite of becoming ill, would still prefer to direct their caring towards others, rather than themselves.

Not Asking But Expecting

Some Earth types find it difficult to ask for what they need and so expect others to read their minds. If others fail, the Earth type may be left disappointed. This is especially the case if they have anticipated other people's needs very well and are doing their best to satisfy them. When they get little back in return a little voice may develop which says, 'What about me?' Neil expressed this very well:

> I sometimes have this hidden agenda. I know what my needs are but it is very hard for people to satisfy them. I tend to expect people to know what they are without me saying. I give out to others then I say, 'Oh, I'm fine', although I know that I'm not. I expect people to go as far as second guessing what I need and I get upset when they don't.

When Earth types can't ask for what they need directly they may express their feelings indirectly. Sometimes this may come out as an angry reaction. They may explode in rage or be continually picking on or resenting other people. They may seem so angry that it may be easy to mistake them for a Wood type. Give them the support and empathy they need, however, and they melt and show us that they are truly an Earth type!

In extreme cases, the Earth type may convince themselves they have no needs. Even when they are given appropriate support and nourishment, they can push it away. Deep inside a part of them may be desperately wanting help and support.

Earth types who feel they are getting no reaction from other people may double their efforts. They may think, 'If I manage to give enough, I'll finally be given something back.' Of course, this rarely works. Carol has already told us about a side of herself which is overly helpful. She also knows that another part reacts in the opposite way.

When I feel well, I have a generosity of spirit to people. When I'm even a little unwell, my generosity of spirit goes. Someone tells me about a problem and I immediately think, 'You call *that* a problem — what about *my* problems?' — but I don't say that.

Some Earth types feel indignant when their generosity doesn't get repaid. It is as if their bank account is empty at the expense of those they have helped. If no one appreciates their 'kindness' their feelings of poverty continue. A cycle has been set up. The Earth types don't ask for what they want and therefore never get their needs met. They may then carry on supporting others. They hope that one day people will appreciate their generosity and helpfulness. Will that 'one day' ever come? As long as their needs are hidden away, it is less likely.

The Earth type who regularly expresses their needs is somewhat different from the person just described.

Expressing Needs a Lot

When we are young, if we don't get what we need, we can complain or make a fuss. Our carers respond. As we grow up, we learn to hold our own spoon, tie our shoelaces and ultimately become independent. Independence, however, is always relative. We are social animals and genuinely depend upon others. There is, nevertheless, an idea of maturity and independence to which we aspire.

One aspect of independence is being flexible about how we get our needs met. If we have a partner who usually prepares our meals, what happens when he or she is sick or away? We might cook our own meals, we might go out to restaurants, we may get friends to give us meals, or we may discover TV dinners. There are options.

Earth types sometimes have difficulty in the transition to independence. Some Earth types feel they don't deserve support or feel they shouldn't ask for things for themselves. Because of this they find it difficult to get help directly. In this case, when they need support, they may go back to the patterns they used when they were young. Many Earth types notice themselves whinging or complaining when their needs are not being taken care of. Jan told us:

> As soon as I get tired I wake up getting whingy and feeling sorry for myself. It's a self-pitying thing. As a child I was told not to whine or I'd be sent to my room so I won't whinge directly and say, 'Oh poor me, please help me.' It's more, 'Oh I'm so tired and I've got this or that to do.' I just whinge on.

When we feel needy we may also feel that we aren't going to be given what is rightly ours. Inga told us:

> I think I have an agenda of, 'It's not fair. I'm not going to get what I need,' or, 'there's not enough for me,' or, 'Oh, what about me?' and a feeling of panic. I kind of harbour resentments if I'm not getting my fair share.

If we feel needy and we aren't getting satisfied, it may be hard for us to stop going on about what we want. We may go into conflict and the part that wants to whinge and complain may be in conflict with the part that has been told not to. Jan said:

> I struggle between being a whinger and not being a whinger. I know someone who, if she has a headache, nobody's had a headache like hers. Someone suggested that I find her difficult to be around because I might not give myself enough time to moan and whinge and I think that's right. If I catch myself I stop, but then I probably complain more at home with my partner.

Of course, these behaviours are not necessarily ones which we experience all the time and many of them can appear only when we are in difficult circumstances. When we are in good health and feel well balanced they might be a less prominent part of our personality. When we feel less well and more tired, they might come more to the fore.

Searching for a Centre

Earth types who didn't feel supported when they were young may later feel that they lack a 'centre'. The lack of centre can be experienced in a variety of ways. It may manifest as a lack of identity or a feeling of instability. Physically, it may be felt as an empty space or weakness in the solar plexus area, but the Earth type does not know what will fill it. Moira used therapy to try and fill the space. She told us:

> I spent a lot of time after I became an adult, trying to develop my centre. I felt I had no centre, just a big hole there, and no one ever filled it. I went to a therapist here and there to try and get something in my centre. I feel it was having a strong sense of myself that I needed.

Others may lose their sense of having a centre in specific situations as Anne explains:

> I had great difficulty when my children left home in being able to say, 'Oh they've gone', and let them go. I definitely lost my centre at that time.

Other Earth types may constantly move from home to home or even from country to country because they have no centre. Without stability inside they may find it hard to settle. For Sandra this went on for a long period of her life:

> I was so uncentred that for years I never lived anywhere for longer than 18 months. By the time I was in my late 30s I knew I had to stop the endless moving around. I'm trying to stay put at the moment. I just hadn't been able to settle.

Over time Earth types may develop a secure centre inside. This allows them to be more settled on the outside. Carol finds she is now more centred in her life:

> I used not to know about my centre at all. Now there's a place of centredness and a still point which I can reach. I've developed a centre-point so I now know I can be positive and not have to do anything or go anywhere — just be a good presence.

In contrast to the person searching for a centre is the Earth type who is a natural homemaker.

Homemaking

Some Earth types love to be at home or on the land. This is not to say that the home and land aren't important to all types. An Earth type, though, can often increase their sense of being centred and grounded when they are at home or looking after the earth. As Jennifer told us:

> For a lot of years I worked as well as bringing up children. I often felt really torn between my home and my career. I thought there was something wrong with me because I enjoyed doing things like tidying the house up and doing housework. Now I accept it's because I am who I am and having a home gives me a centre. I love to have a day off during the week where I can potter around and that's actually meeting some of my needs.

For a long time Carol did the opposite to Jennifer. She soon discovered that she needed a quality home too:

> I used to make my home circumstances poor because there are some other people who are poor. I'd live in a hovel to kind of resonate with poor people. I learnt later that home and nurturing allows us to do the things we value. I now have a warm easy going home and it makes me feel content.

Other Earth types find looking after a garden or being on the Earth can be beneficial. By being on the land they're literally in their element. Karen said:

> I have a concern for the Earth and can connect to the Earth. We manage 20 acres of land as a wildlife reserve, it's full of birds and it's wonderful. I get a lot of positive feedback about it. I also use gardening as a way of grounding myself and I find it very calming.

The earth itself can be an important source of nourishment for an Earth type. The Chinese visualized people standing with their heads in the Heavens and their feet on the ground. The feet on the ground is a sign of being earthed and being 'down to earth' and practical.

By standing on the Earth with our feet apart and our legs slightly bent we can allow the earth energies to enter our bodies through our feet. The extra connection to the earth which we gain from this simple stance can be very healing and it can also enable us to experience ourselves as more secure, balanced and centred inside. There is a great emphasis in the Chinese exercise called Tai Chi Chuan of being able to be firmly rooted through your legs. For more on this, see the exercises for Earth types.

Many Earth types can find themselves disheartened by what they now see happening to the Earth. This matter may be of concern to all types for different reasons. For Earth types the issues are mostly around the Earth as a provider. Realizing that the earth can no longer provide us with high quality nourishment can make us very insecure. Neil said:

Ecological things are important to me and they make me very upset and angry. The state of the planet and seeing the earth becoming polluted. But I find myself getting stuck and not being able to do anything about it.

VIRTUES AND VICES OF AN EARTH TYPE

Depending on the health of the Earth type, these strategies produce both virtues and vices. Some of the virtues are:
♦ The ability to give support and care for others
♦ The ability to put others before themselves
♦ Love of the family and homemaking
♦ Love and care for food
♦ An affinity to the earth.
Some of the vices are:
♦ Over-nourishing others when they don't need or want it
♦ Not asking for support when they need it and neglecting themselves
♦ Getting whingy when they don't get what they want
♦ Obsessing and worrying needlessly
♦ Being unable to think clearly.

A FAMOUS EARTH TYPE — DIANA, PRINCESS OF WALES

Princess Diana was in some ways a typical Earth type and it was many of her Earth characteristics which brought her close to so many people's hearts. She exhibited the strengths of the Earth type by her gift for highlighting the needs of the most neglected victims of society such as those with Aids, leprosy and other serious illnesses. She also supported vulnerable people such as the homeless, sick children and the disabled. Like many other Earth types who mother and care for others she found that visiting people who were unwell was a healing experience both for them and herself.

The choice of the cause that became her crusade towards the end of her life was one we could almost have predicted — landmines — bombs hidden in the earth and which cause much harm and distress to humanity.

The princess could be said to have a combination of strategies. She was caring and mothering, and a homemaker. At the same time she could also be quite needy. She was passionate about her family and loved her boys — she had a great sense of fun as well as being protective of their needs. At the same time she understood the need to keep them down to earth and in touch with the suffering of the world. She took them with her to see refuges for the homeless. She didn't want them to take the privileged life they led for granted.

Like many Earth types much of her sensitivity to others undoubtedly arose through her own childhood insecurities. When she was still a child her parents underwent a traumatic divorce and she lost her mother. When she was young she must have had some extremely lonely and insecure times with few people to turn to.

We also know that for a long period the eating disorder bulimia — a problem for many Earth types — made havoc of her life. She spent long periods feeling desperate for help from those around her — especially her husband Prince Charles. Not surprisingly, he neither understood nor found it possible to meet her needs. We are told that the more she felt neglected and ignored the more she would try to draw attention to herself and try to get sympathy. She is even reported to have fallen down the stairs on purpose and cut her wrists so that those around her would take notice.

Princess Diana was loved and respected for her ability to nourish and care for others who were in need. She also revealed to us that even a princess has the need for support and help. She had experienced human suffering and distress like the rest of us. She showed us clearly the conflicts and insecurities which an Earth type can face. Although she hadn't fully resolved her problems, it was clear that she had worked to resolve them and that she had grown in confidence through this process.

GOLDEN RULES FOR EARTH TYPES

♦ From the viewpoint of eternity, others' needs and your own are equal.
♦ Discriminate whose needs are important and when.
♦ Think less about what you want and more about what you need.
♦ When you nourish yourself with wisdom and care, you nourish the divine inside you.
♦ Assume you carry another's heart within you and act accordingly.

Notes

1   Weiger, L, 1965: *Chinese Characters*; page 209.
2   Larre, Claude and Rochat de la Vallee, Elisabeth (trans), 1987: *The Secret Treatise of the Spiritual Orchid*; pages 97–101.
3   Goleman, Daniel: *Emotional Intelligence*; Bloomsbury Publishing, Chapter 7, page 100.
4   Davis Spiegel et al: 'Effect of Psychological Treatment on Survival of Patients with Metastatic Breast Cancer'; published by the *Lancet* Number 8668, 1989.

Chapter 7

EXERCISES FOR EARTH TYPES

INTRODUCTION

The exercises in this chapter are aimed at enabling Earth types to find a better emotional balance. Some useful goals for an Earth type are:

♦ To break their cycle of worrying
♦ To separate their own needs from the needs of other people
♦ To learn to accept and respect their own needs and develop mature ways of satisfying them
♦ To channel their natural need to care for others in ways that are truly productive and useful to others
♦ To develop a feeling or sense of being centred and grounded.

USING THE EXERCISES

We suggest that you read an exercise through before you start it. All of the exercises are laid out in a similar style. Following the *introduction*, we tell you approximately *how long* it will take to complete. Obviously some of you will take more time and others less. The exercises are then divided into stages. They start with:

♦ the *purpose* of the exercise and then
♦ the *process* or the steps of the exercise.

The theme of each step is in bold so that you have a summary. At the end of some exercises we have a section called *'matters arising'*. Here we discuss issues which could come up while you do the exercise.

THE EXERCISES FOR EARTH TYPES

+ Points of view — objective, other and self
+ The objective point of view
+ Experiencing another person's point of view
+ My own point of view
+ Creating a balanced point of view
+ The people I care for
+ Dissolving your worries
+ Qigong exercise — reaching heaven and earth
+ Qigong exercise — grounding ourselves

EXERCISE 1 POINTS OF VIEW — OBJECTIVE, OTHER AND SELF

General introduction

The first three exercises for Earth types help us to experience the world from different points of view. These exercises have been adapted to suit the Earth type's special needs.

A change in point of view can radically alter the way we experience things. For example, when two people are in the middle of a stressful and difficult situation they may change their perspective when one of them says, 'You know, five years from now we'll look back on this and laugh.'

Johanna is an Earth type. Both at work and at home she tended to be thinking of other people's welfare rather than her own. Just learning to go to the three points of view made a big difference to her. She said:

I always assumed I knew what others wanted, but I found that I could be wrong. Deep inside though a part of me really did know as I discovered through doing this exercise. The other big difference is how unfamiliar it was to ask myself, 'What do I, Joanna, want right now?' That has been strange. And very good for me.

There are many different points of view, but the three main ones[1] are: The 'Objective-position', the 'Other-position' and the 'Self-position'. Here is a little bit about each of them:

The *Objective point of view* is where we are looking at both ourselves and another person as if we were an impartial observer. This position can lead to wise observations, but if we only take up this position we will have very little engagement in life.

The *Other person's point of view* is when we step into the other's shoes and see the situation and ourselves from their point of view. This position can lead us to thinking about other people's needs, but if we only take up this position we will neglect our own needs.

The *Self point of view* is when we are firmly rooted in ourselves and are seeing things clearly from our own point of view. This can lead us to knowing our own needs, but if we only take up this position we will become selfish with little wisdom and no real awareness of others' needs or experience.[2]

A well balanced person will tend to move flexibly from one position to another as the situation demands. These exercises will enable you to take an 'Objective' or 'Outside Position' which can then be used to balance the first two points of view. These three exercises may take time to do and can be done in stages. They are root exercises and will be most useful when repeated, so as to develop greater internal flexibility.

We will describe how to do these exercises using three chairs. You may find it easiest to actually change positions as you do it. You can do it without chairs if you prefer. The 'self' and 'other' positions should face each other. The objective observer should sit facing both positions (see Figure 15).

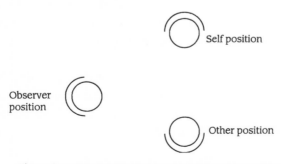

Self position

Observer position

Other position

Figure 7: POSITIONS OF CHAIRS FOR DIFFERENT POINTS OF VIEW

EXERCISE 1a — THE OBJECTIVE POINT OF VIEW

Purpose

Taking up an objective point of view allows us to discover our already existing, natural abilities. We can also find out valuable information about ourselves and others. Earth types can get overwhelmed by their own emotions. This exercise will help them to separate from them and gain a new perspective. The objective point of view is sometimes called the perspective of the 'neutral observer' or even the 'wise person'.

Time needed: At first, 10–15 minutes. Later you will be much quicker.

Process

1 **Pick a person or situation you wish to understand.** This may be a difficulty which is not turning out as you want it to, or a person you don't understand. It is best if some new insights or perceptions would be useful.

2 **Prepare some helpful questions.** Write these down as if you are detached from yourself. For example, if your name is Ann and you want to know about an interaction between you and Paul you might ask:

   ♦ What does Ann (you) want and what does Paul (the other significant person) want?

   ♦ What is going on between these two?

   ♦ What is stopping progress?

   ♦ Is there something Ann does not know but should?

   ♦ What is the best way for Ann to act?

3 **Put yourself in the objective point of view.** Imagine that you and this person are going through the situation you have chosen. As a neutral observer sit facing them. In your imagination they can be sitting in chairs facing each other (see Figure 7). Alternatively, they can be in any other position that is appropriate.

4 **Now adjust your perspective.** Notice the people in your image. Adjust them so that they are similar in size, distance and clarity. If there are any voices adjust them so that they come from whoever is speaking.

   Refer to each person in the scene by their names or by the pronouns 'she' or 'he'. You might look at your image of each person separately and say, 'This is Ann' (your name) and then, 'This is Paul.' (the other person's name).

5   **Now, adjust your feelings.** When watching and listening to these two, notice how you feel. As an observer you might have feelings of curiosity or compassion. You should not, however, be experiencing Ann's feelings. Ask yourself if these are the feelings of you as an observer or if they are they still your own (Ann's) feelings. If they are your own feelings, simply ask them to move from you (the objective person) to Ann in the image you have. You might say to yourself:

♦ 'I allow these feelings to move to Ann where they belong.'

Now check that they are there. By doing this you are keeping the observer position clear.

Your adjustment of the image so far is designed to develop your capacity for objectivity. You may achieve it the first time — it may well take longer.

6   **Now ask the questions from step 2.** Go back to your adjusted image, and ask the questions. Whatever answers you get, note them down. You are discovering the wisdom that lies within yourself.

This is as far as we go right now with the Objective-position. You may have found the process easy or difficult. You can continue to the next stage or take as long as you need to master the adjustments described in steps 3 to 6.

EXERCISE 1b — EXPERIENCING ANOTHER PERSON'S POINT OF VIEW

Purpose

This exercise allows us to step into another person's shoes and see a situation from their point of view. At times an Earth type may only notice their own needs and fail to notice how others are feeling. The next exercise is to increase our ability to see things from our own perspective. We will then learn to balance our own and other's points of view.

Time needed: 10–15 minutes.

Process

1   **Find a recent incident.** This could be one where you are helping someone else, but you have other demands placed on you at the same time. It could also be one where someone else wants something from you and you are reluctant to agree. Alternatively, it may be one where your needs and

another person's needs are in conflict and some new insights would be helpful.

2 **Study the other person.** Place two chairs opposite each other (see Figure 15). Sit on the 'Self' chair and look at the other person. Remember their posture, gestures, voice tone and facial expression in as much detail as you can. Remember whatever else is relevant, for example, their age, experience, abilities, health, problems, relationships and needs. 'Relevant' means what their connection with you is and anything that would help you to understand their needs.

3 **Now change chairs and sit in the chair of the 'Other' position to step into the other person's point of view.** In your imagination go back to the time you were with them in the incident you identified above. To do this see what they are seeing and hear what they are hearing. Look at yourself in the opposite chair exactly as they saw you at the time. This is a complex task and you may do it immediately and it may take you a while. Here are some ways to help you to get into the other person's position:

♦ Take up the posture, gestures and/or facial expression they had at the time.
♦ Talk as they are talking, saying the same kinds of words and in a similar tone of voice.
♦ Imagine their body is your body.
♦ If your name is 'Ann', and their name is 'Paul', you can say to yourself, 'I am Paul and I am with Ann who is over there.'
♦ Imagine what they felt like at the time and let yourself feel that way.

If this takes you a while, remind yourself that you are developing a very useful skill and persist. You will not do this perfectly. Going through these steps allows you closely to observe the person and find out what it's like to be him or her.

4 **Now gather some information about this person.** Find out how this person feels, how they are experiencing you and what they want. You might gather these by staying in their position and saying:

♦ 'I am feeling ...'
♦ 'I am feeling ... about Ann — I think ... about Ann.'
♦ 'What I really want right now is ...'
♦ 'What is important to me in this situation is ...'

5 **Come back to yourself.** A word of warning. If you are extremely good at this task you will have to make especially sure that you are no longer taking the position of this person. If this is difficult, deliberately think of something else, stand up and shake yourself or jump around.

6   **As yourself, describe to yourself what you learned.** Write down what you now know about this other person which you did not know before. Ask yourself how you might use this new information.

EXERCISE 1c — MY OWN POINT OF VIEW

Purpose

The 'Self-position' is when you are firmly rooted in yourself and are seeing the world clearly from your own point of view. Some readers may assume that Self-position is an easy position to take up. This is not always true and many Earth types find that it is easier to empathize with other people's viewpoints than their own. A failure to be fully grounded in our own point of view (at least some of the time), can lead to self-neglect. Self-position involves clarity about who we are and what we want in a situation.
   Time needed: 10–15 minutes.

Process

1   **As in the previous exercise, find a recent incident**. You can use the same incident from the previous exercise. It could be one where you were helping someone else, but perhaps you had other demands on you at the same time. Another could be where someone else wanted something from you and you were very reluctant to agree. It should involve at least one other person and possibly more. Choose what would be typical of your everyday life.
2   **Imagine the incident again, from your own point of view.**
3   **Now, pay attention to your picture(s) and what you are seeing.** Sit in the chair for yourself and see the other person in front of you. Adjust your image and see the other person according to the following criteria. She/he is:
   ♦ Directly in front of you
   ♦ At a comfortable distance. Adjust the distance between the chairs so that you do not feel overwhelmed or out of touch. Be at a distance where you have good contact
   ♦ Now make sure that you are fully in your own body, not slightly to the side or back, but immediately within yourself. See the other person from this position. If you seem to be even a small amount out of alignment within yourself make an adjustment.

4 **Now consider and possibly adjust the sounds in your image.** If there are no sounds include what they are or might be. Adjust the sounds in the following ways:

♦ Notice the tones and relative volumes of the different voices.

♦ Notice if your voice comes from your throat and if not, ensure it does.

♦ Notice if the voice of the other(s) comes from them and if not, adjust your hearing so that the sound does come from its real source.

♦ Is there any commentary or inner voice and where is that located?

♦ If there is a commentary or internal voice, then experiment with moving it, e.g. if it is in the left ear, move it to the right, but leave it wherever it feels natural.

5 **Now, use language to confirm this point of view.** Refer to the other person as 'he' or 'she' or 'them' or by their individual name. Say something like, 'There is Paul and I am here (or this is me)'.

6 **Now, check and, if relevant, adjust your feelings.** When watching and listening to the other(s), notice how you are feeling. Even if your feelings seem straightforward and understandable, ask yourself if these are *your* feelings. If they are not, you may know whose feelings they are. Say to yourself, 'I allow these feelings to return to whoever they belong to.' When you are comfortable that the only feelings you have are your own, confirm this by saying to yourself, 'These are my feelings.'

7 **When you are fully in your Self-position, ask the following questions:**

♦ Do I feel comfortable here and if not, why? (You may need to ask once again if all the feelings you are having are your own — step 6 above.)

♦ What do I want right now?

♦ What else?

The final two questions may change your feelings and, if so, you can cycle back to step 6.

EXERCISE 2 — CREATING A BALANCED POINT OF VIEW

Introduction

Emily was a primary school teacher and was worn out from caring for others. She cared for the students, she cared for other teachers and she cared for her husband and two teenage sons. She said that 'life's not worth living if you don't help others'. At the same time she was exhausted and was considering going to the doctor to see if he thought she had ME.

In the following exercise, she had an opportunity to consider the connection between caring for herself and caring for others. She ended up using the statement in step 6 as a 'mantra' which she would repeat over and over to herself because it had such a positive effect. A big discovery, she says, was that her sons benefited when she didn't 'care' so much for them. Two months after first doing the exercise, she says the changes are still taking place.

Time needed: 10–20 minutes

Purpose

This exercise encourages us to be flexible in our ability to move in and out of the Objective, Other and Self points of view. Emotional stability and richness come from being able to move between these viewpoints. Getting stuck in any one of the three points of view or having a distorted way of gaining access to them will limit us. If we practise moving in and out of the three positions, we will become flexible at doing so.

Process

1 **Find a situation involving yourself and someone else.** The person you choose should be typical of the 'others' in your life. This could be more than one person, but it will be easier if you have one. You may wish to use the same examples as the ones used in the previous exercises.

2 **In sequence, take up the Observer-position, the Other-position and the Self-position.** Do this more rapidly this time. Change chairs as you do so. Assess which position is the easiest for you, which is the least easy and which is in between. Resolve to practise the position you find the least easy.

3 **Now take up the position of a very wise person or your higher self.** To do this go back to the chair of the 'Objective-position'. If the two people involved are Ann (yourself) and Paul, then say out loud, 'The needs of Ann are important and equal in importance to those of Paul. The needs of Paul are important and equal to those of Ann.'

If saying this statement brings up new feelings, take a few moments to acknowledge them. Return to the objective position and repeat the statement again. Continue repeating this statement until you are comfortable with it. If you cannot feel comfortable while saying the statement, that is fine.

4 **From the same position as in 3 above, say out loud,** 'Ann is responsible for caring for herself and if she does, this means she can receive care from others. Paul is responsible for caring for himself and if he does, this means he can receive care from others.' If saying this statement generates new feelings, take a few moments to acknowledge them.

5 **Now change chairs again to the 'Self' position chair and say,** 'My needs are important and I take responsibility for caring for myself. This means I can accept care from others and I can care for others.' Again, if saying this statement brings up new feelings, take a few moments to acknowledge them. Continue repeating this statement until you are comfortable. If you cannot feel comfortable while saying the statement, that is fine. When you move through the whole exercise again, you will find you feel different.

6 **Once more, in sequence, take up the Observer-position, the Other-position and the Self-position.** Come out of the exercise, and ask yourself:

   ♦ How am I feeling right now?
   ♦ How am I different from before the exercise?

Write down any changes in your notebook.

EXERCISE 3 — THE PEOPLE I CARE FOR

Introduction

Viv, like many Earth types, found it easier to look after other people rather than herself. She cared for her mother-in-law who was terminally ill; she cared for her aromatherapy patients; and she cared for her two teenage daughters. She was brave and felt upset when she wondered about who was supposed to care for her.

The following exercise helped Viv both understand why no one seemed to care for her (at least in the way she wanted) and how to get the care she wanted. Six weeks on she said she was in transition, getting more of the caring she wanted and occasionally slipping back into, what she now called, 'my martyr's habits'.

Time needed: 10–15 minutes.

Purpose

This exercise is for those who find it easier to direct their caring energy to others rather than themselves. The purpose is to help you discover what stops you caring well for yourself and then to find a process whereby you give yourself your fair share of the caring love and energy. You do not have to be a selfless martyr to benefit from this exercise — many of us need a gentle push to direct some of our caring energy to ourselves. It is fine to do this exercise in two stages, up to step 4 and then step 5 to 6.

Process

1 **Think of a person for whom you do a lot of caring**. The caring can be in your personal or professional life.
2 **Find out 'how you think' about this person.** To do this imagine that this person is in front of you. Notice your image of the person and check the following areas:
   ♦ Where do you see the person — straight in front of you, to the left or to the right?
   ♦ Do you see the person at eye level, above or below?
   ♦ Is the picture moving or still, black and white or in colour, is the person face/half-body or full body?
   ♦ How far away is the picture?
   ♦ Do you hear the person's voice and if so from where?

   Make some notes about how you represent this person. For instance, the picture may be straight in front of you, at eye level, have slight movement in it, be in full colour and be about three feet away. The person in the picture may be speaking.
3 **Now, put yourself in the 'cared for place'.** Imagine yourself in the same way as you imagined the person(s) you care for. Use the notes you made in the previous step to adjust your image of yourself so that it has the characteristics you discovered in step 2.
4 **Let yourself know you are worth caring for.** If you feel comfortable, looking at yourself in the 'cared for' place, then simply say, 'You are worth being cared for. Which means I am worth caring for.' Notice how you feel saying that.

   Hold this image for a moment or two and notice what feelings arise. If feelings do arise, just hold the image and the feelings. Allow them both to be. If you can't hold the image, then just allow the feelings to be. If you can't put yourself in that place, then go back to your image of the person you care for and slip yourself into the same place.

   A response some people have to the image of themselves in the 'cared for' space is that they couldn't be cared for in the way that they like to care for others. It may be unimaginable or there may be some negative feelings around being needy. This perception may be accompanied by hurt or tearful feelings. If this happens, **just allow the feelings to release** — these feelings are blocking you from caring equally for yourself. Take whatever time you need to do this.

5 **When you are comfortable with putting yourself in the position you reserve for those you care for, ask the following questions.** The following assumes your name is Ann:

♦ What are Ann's main needs right now?
♦ How can she best get them met?
♦ Does she need to ask for help from someone and if so whom?

People describe their needs in various ways. In answer to the first question you may say, 'I have a need for X', where X is, for example, care, understanding, someone to listen to me, someone to talk to, physical rest, a better diet, acknowledgement, physical stroking, loving attention, public respect, being taken seriously, or information about what is going on.

6 **Determine what you have received from this exercise and how to proceed.**

This is an exercise which you may wish to make part of your everyday life. Once you know the process, take a moment to put yourself in the appropriate place and ask, 'What does she or he need right now?' When you discover what you need, act promptly. If you find yourself saying that you can never have it, confirm that you need it and trust your natural intelligence to help you. Do this short 'check into your needs' three times a day for two weeks and notice the benefits.

EXERCISE 4 — DISSOLVING YOUR WORRIES

Introduction

Raymond had a habit of just worrying. When asked what he worried about he smiled and said, 'Well, anything.' What he meant by worrying was thinking about small things like getting to an appointment on time or whether one of his clients would actually turn up to a meeting — things he had planned for and couldn't do anything more about — and going over and over them in his mind. He described the following exercise as a 'blessing' and said it took about two weeks to replace his 'worry' with the process described here.

Time needed: 10–20 minutes.

Purpose

The purpose of this exercise is to turn a worry habit into one that checks the validity of the worry and replaces the worry with a more positive and optimistic state. This exercise is designed for the small worries where you know that it would really be better to let the worry go.

Process

1 **Think of something which is worrying you or if you have more than one worry write down a list.** The nature of a worry is that we sometimes imagine an event as if it has already happened. Your list may look something like this:
   ♦ I'll do something stupid at the party tonight
   ♦ My child might have an accident
   ♦ I don't think I'll be able to cope with the work I'm doing at present
   ♦ I might fall off the ladder when I clean the windows
2 **Take one of your worries and notice what image it creates in your head, any thoughts you have with the picture and any feelings it creates.** For example, if you think you might do something stupid at the party tonight you may imagine a party going on in front of you and hear other people saying, 'Isn't she stupid'. You might at the same time feel a tightness in your stomach.
3 **Ask yourself, 'Is this worry useful for me?'** If the answer is 'Yes' then ask, 'How is it useful?' For instance, if you worry about your child having an accident, this may have a positive function for you and cause you to make her or his environment safe. Write down how your worry is useful. Make a note if the answer is 'No'.
4 **Now place an imaginary frame around the image of your worry.** At the same time keep what you felt and heard associated with the picture. For example, if you are imagining the party then you will see the party taking place in a framed picture and still hear the words and feel the tightness in your stomach.
5 **Now get an image of yourself having coped with your worry in a positive way.** See yourself as if the situation has taken place and you have

dealt with it well. If it is an ongoing situation see it as if you are coping well with it.

When forming this new image, bear in mind your reason for having the worry. For example, if you worry about your child having an accident then see yourself being aware of her or his safety needs but also that you are coping well. See yourself looking calm and relaxed or feeling any other positive feelings associated with this image. Hear any positive words. For instance you may hear yourself saying, 'I coped well tonight'. *This image should make you feel good*. Place this positive image in a frame.

7 **Shrink the positive image.** Now in your mind, shrink the positive image and place it in the corner of the original image you had when you were worrying.

8 **Make the small positive image grow rapidly larger,** replacing the image you have of worrying which recedes and gets smaller. Repeat this 5 times always starting with the 'worry-image' large and the new positive image small and allowing the positive image to replace the worry image. It is important to do this rapidly. You might even say, 'Whooooosh' as you do it to emphasize the rapid movement.

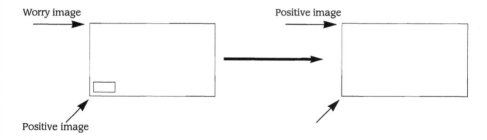

Worry image

Positive image

Positive image

Figure 8: A WORRY IMAGE CHANGING TO A POSITIVE IMAGE

Go back and try to find your original worry. It might well have disappeared! You may want to do this exercise with another worry.[3]

QIGONG EXERCISES FOR EARTH TYPES

Introduction

Martin is an Earth type who thought he should, but never did exercise. He was attracted by the idea of using his mind and imagination to move his energy in a

Qigong exercise. For him, the result of doing these two exercises regularly was that he felt much better in his body. In particular, he said that he 'regained his legs' even though he hadn't noticed that somehow he had been feeling his legs less and less.

Time needed: Five minutes per day building to ten minutes

Purpose

Both of these exercises will help to strengthen the energy of an Earth type. It is best to do them every day, or at least five days a week.

QIGONG EXERCISE FOR REACHING HEAVEN AND EARTH

Process

1 **Stand with your feet shoulders' width apart and the inside edges of your feet parallel.** From your hips, bounce gently up and down, no more than an inch or so. Feel how your weight travels down from your hips to your feet which are solid on the floor.

   Notice any differences between your legs and any feelings of discomfort, heaviness or thickness. Allow your arms to hang by your sides with your palms turned slightly outwards so your armpits feel open.

2 **Hold an imaginary ball in front of you.** Move your hands so that your left hand is palm up and in front of you, just below your navel, and your right hand is palm down and in front of your solar plexus (see Figure 17). Relax your shoulders and whole body and hold this ball for a few moments. Your hands should feel as if the ball is a real one.

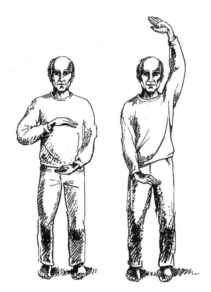

Figure 9: QIGONG EXERCISE FOR REACHING HEAVEN AND EARTH

3 **Move your hands closer together.** Bring the left up and lower the right. Let them pass each other. The right hand continues down until it is pushing downwards, the wrist bent backwards, right in front of your groin. At the same time, the left hand raises up, turns over at about chest height and ends up with the palm pushing upwards and the wrist bent backwards above your head. Ideally, the hands arrive in these positions at the same time. Hold this position for a few moments and enjoy the stretch. If you feel any pain, adjust so that you can stretch as much as you can, but without pain.

4 **Now, exchange the position of the hands.** Turn the palms towards each other and let them return to hold a ball in the same position as before. Now continue their movement past each other, as in step 3, but in the opposite direction. You will end up with your right hand, palm upwards, pushing to the sky above your head, and the left hand pushing into the earth in front of your groin. Continue slowly exchanging the hands, feeling your abdomen, arms and hands as you move.

5 **When you know the movement, coordinate your breathing.** Breathe in as your hands come closer together and breathe out as they push one up and one down. Ideally, the outbreath should be longer. This will correspond with taking a moment to stretch when your arms are fully extended.

6   **To finish**, simply hold the ball in front of you for one breath and return your hands to your sides. Notice any differences you feel in your body and in your feelings.[4]

QIGONG EXERCISE FOR GROUNDING OURSELVES

Process

1   **Stand with your feet shoulders' width apart and your knees slightly bent.** Stand with the inside edges of your feet parallel. From your hips, bounce gently up and down, no more than an inch or so. Feel how your weight travels down from your hips to your feet which are solid on the floor. Notice any differences between each of your legs and any feelings of discomfort, heaviness or thickness. Allow your arms to hang by your sides with your palms turned slightly outwards so your armpits feel open.

2   **Let your weight move slowly from one foot to the other.** Move first to the left and then to the right. Feel, as it were, inside the leg and notice any tight, blocked or 'thick' areas. Do this for a minute or two.

3   **Begin to raise one foot an inch or two off the ground and then the other, back and forth.** You will probably be moving back and forth more quickly now, but still notice the different feelings in each leg as you did in stage 2. Do this for a minute or two. If your mind wanders, just bring it back to your legs and scan in more detail. Ask yourself: 'What are the feelings in the feet, the ankles, the calf, the knee, the thigh and the hips?' And then ask in more detail: 'What about the front part of my foot? What about the arch of my foot?' and so on.

4   **At this point you may, or you may not, like to have a 'stomp'** which is simply letting go and running on the spot but really concentrating on the foot contacting the earth.

5   **Reverse the order of the movements.** If you had a stomp, go back to stage 3, then stage 2 and then stage 1. If you did not stomp, go back to stage 2 and then stage 1. When you are just standing, again notice how your legs compared to how they were at the beginning of the exercise. Also notice if your abdomen and head are any clearer. Repeat this exercise regularly and over time notice how your legs feel different.

Notes

1   Dilts, Robert B; 1994; pages 279–80.

2   There are many sources of the perceptual positions within the NLP literature, but for the details of alignment, we are particularly indebted to: Andreas, Connirae; 1994.

3   See Bandler, Richard, 1985: *Using Your Brain — For a Change;* pages 131–52. This chapter describes the basic 'swish' process which is used in the worry exercise. The swish process itself has many other uses.

4   There are many sources of this exercise in the Qigong literature, but this exercise can be found in: Yang, Jwing-Ming, 1996, second edition; pages 50–51.

Chapter 8

THE METAL TYPE - RESPECTING OURSELVES

JOAN IS A METAL TYPE

'I seem to have spent my whole life looking for something, but I still feel as if it's missing,' Joan told us. She admits that she's achieved a great deal in her life and she looks forward to celebrating her fiftieth birthday soon. She is a mother of three and a grandmother. She has a PhD in psychology and works as a clinical psychologist.

Joan is a Metal type and has a white facial colour. As she speaks her voice catches slightly as if she might cry. This is called a 'weeping' voice. Grief is the emotion associated with this Element and although Joan has not been 'bereaved', the feeling that there is 'something missing' is a similar sense of loss.

This grief is something she experiences every day. 'I don't talk much about my feelings,' she says, 'and I'm certainly not the type to wear my heart on my sleeve — that would be too gross. If I had to describe how I feel though I'd say that I feel an ache or a sort of longing feeling in my chest. I always think I could do things better.'

Joan's special commitment is to Tai Chi Chuan — gentle Chinese exercises which she practises daily and also teaches. 'I would like to improve my Tai Chi as I never feel I do it well enough. One teacher I've seen can actually move people with his energy. I'd like to do something like that — it would prove to me I could really do it'.

Ask her students about her and it's a different story. They hold her in awe. One says, 'We all admire her and she does really know her stuff! She's almost unworldly and seems detached from the everyday things of life.' Joan admits that she sometimes has this affect on people. 'I know that sometimes people think I'm perfect — I'd hate to show them the real me. I'm really quite fragile inside. I'd like to live up to what they think about me but inside I feel I'm sadly lacking. That's why I'm trying so hard to improve in everything I do. I've done lots of different things in my life but they're all to the same end — finding something meaningful.'

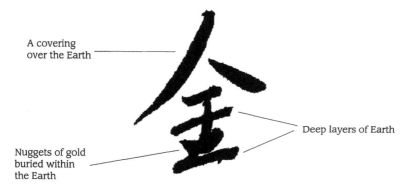

A covering over the Earth

Deep layers of Earth

Nuggets of gold buried within the Earth

Figure 10: THE CHINESE CHARACTER FOR METAL

THE METAL ELEMENT IN NATURE

The character for Metal is Jin (drawn above). It includes the character for Earth (see chapter 6, page 103). The Earth character normally has only a base horizontal line and one other. The Metal character, however, has an extra horizontal line. This indicates many layers deep within the Earth. This character has a sloping roof on top, signifying something covered over. The two shorter lines symbolize nuggets of gold buried deep within the Earth. The whole character describes something small in quantity, but of great value and buried deep within the earth.[1]

Many elemental systems have been created, but only the Chinese included a Metal Element. This Element was named well before the birth of Christ — before we had steel mills, aluminium production and many of the precious metals we use today. So what is the meaning of Metal to the Chinese?

Gold, which is the most precious metal, is described in the Chinese character for Metal. We can also think of Metal as the minerals or trace elements in the Earth or in our food. Ninety-six per cent of our body is made up of carbohydrates, protein, fat and vitamins. The remaining four per cent is made from minerals which are used to regulate and balance our body chemistry. Often these minerals are required in amounts referred to as traces. For example, a person may require

400 or more grams of carbohydrate a day, but less than a millionth of that amount of chromium. Yet chromium is every bit as essential. The highly valued Metal is deeply buried within.

The Chinese also described the sky as an inverted Metal bowl and the stars as holes in that bowl. Our Lungs draw in energy from the Heavens (or the sky) and thus a link was made between air, Metal and the breath of life.

Metal can be thought of as those small but essential materials which, if missing, deplete the quality of the whole. It can also be described as the invisible air without which our vitality immediately suffers.

THE BACKGROUND TO METAL IN CHINESE MEDICINE

Introduction

The Metal Element consists of the notion of Metal itself — as expressed in the character — and all the Metal associations. The key associations are:

Organs   Lung and Large Intestine
Spirit   P'o — the mental-spiritual aspect of the Metal Element
Colour   White
Sound   Weeping
Emotion   Grief
Odour   Rotten

The discussion of these associations will help us recognize Metal types and, in particular, to understand the connections between the Organ functions and the mental processes described later.

The Lung

Chinese medicine tells us that the Lungs 'receive Qi energy from the Heavens' and also 'govern respiration'. Physically this is through breathing. In a broader sense, it is the capacity to 'take things in' mentally and spiritually. We will discuss this taking-in process more deeply later in the chapter.

Proper breathing allows us to maintain sufficient levels of energy. Most of us understand that if we breathe shallowly we will not take in our full share of vital energy. If the Lungs are impaired, we can consciously breathe more deeply. This will temporarily compensate but without the deliberate, longer-term exercise, a person's basic energy will remain low.

The Lung and Defensive Qi

The Lung also has the function of spreading or dispersing what is called 'Defensive' or 'Protective' Qi all over the body. This Defensive Qi lies just under the skin. Chinese medicine tells us that it protects us from climatic conditions such as wind, cold and damp. If these conditions penetrate through the Defensive Qi they could result in infections and achy joints. Someone with weak Lungs might have a poor resistance to catching colds and flus and be more likely to have allergic responses to the increasing pollution in our atmosphere.

The Mental-Spiritual Aspect of the Lungs

The mental-spiritual aspect of the Lungs is the 'P'o' or physical soul. The P'o has two relevant functions. The first function is similar to the 'Defensive Qi' referred to above. On a physical level the Lungs give us the ability to ward off infections like coughs and colds. Because the Lungs are vulnerable to these 'attacks' by infections they are called the 'fragile' Organ. On a mental and spiritual level we are correspondingly fragile. People who have weak Lungs will almost always be open to emotional or psychic assault. This is often hidden by the fact that they appear to cope well and be very competent in many areas of their lives.

A second function is the capacity to have clear sensations. A strong P'o means that our physical sensations — of vision, sound and body — are keen which in turn allows us to be physically alert and animated. The Chinese say that someone has 'P'o Li' when they have high spirits which leads them to become vigorously involved in an activity.

The Large Intestine

The Large Intestine is sometimes called 'the Drainer of the Dregs'. This is because it removes all waste products from the system via a bowel action. The Lungs and Large Intestine have opposing but complementary functions. The Lungs are responsible for taking in pure energy and the Large Intestines for letting go of impurities.

People with an imbalance in their Large Intestine may physically have bowel problems but they can also be affected mentally and spiritually. An imbalance of the Large Intestine energy might result in people retaining physical waste products or, on another level, holding onto unhealthy feelings or thoughts. The Metal type may hold onto the past instead of letting go and moving on. Carol, a Metal type describes how this affects her:

Letting go is difficult about some personal issues — stuff to do with relationships. I might have decided to forget something but then I still think 'What if ...' and keep thinking about the past.

THESE SYMPTOMS MAY ARISE WHEN THE LUNGS AND LARGE INTESTINE ARE WEAK OR OBSTRUCTED

Some of these symptoms are more physical and some more mental or of the spirit. Chinese medicine being 'energetic' did not make this an important distinction.

Shortness of breath, a weak voice and a dislike of speaking. Daytime sweating. Easily catches colds. Over-sensitive or vulnerable to outside criticism. Coughing, a hoarse voice, a dry mouth and throat. Difficulty dealing with loss. Tiredness. Constipation or diarrhoea.

Observable Signs of a Metal Type

The following are some key signs which indicate that a person is a Metal type:

♦ A white almost shiny colour on the face — especially around the eyes, but also around the mouth and in the laugh lines
♦ A body odour for which the English translation is 'rotten'. This odour feels quite dense, tingles inside the nose, and seems to penetrate the nostrils. It is sometimes described as the odour of meat which is going off.
♦ A weeping sound in the voice where the ends of sentences or phrases tend to tail off and it is almost as if the speaker could begin to cry.
♦ The person's emotional expression, which we will deal with in a later section.

Posture, Gestures and Facial Expression

The face and body of a Metal type will often, although not necessarily, show indications of chronic grief or loss. Acute grief might well manifest in tears and wailing. Chronic grief, which results from an ongoing sense of loss, will manifest in slack cheek and jaw muscles with deficient tone.

The breathing of a Metal type may also be shallow. For moments it may even appear to have stopped. Sometimes the chest may look underdeveloped, collapsed or inert. Marion, a Metal type, told us:

> My chest is small and narrow and I have small shoulders. It's a weak area. I have endless chest problems. As a child I always had colds which became a cough.

Another characteristic of a Metal type which is frequently observed comes from a strategy described later as 'distancing'. Metal types can be present, even alert, but internally withdrawn. This protects them from perceived external threats. The face is still and the eyes alert but the person behind the face does not respond to psychological stimuli. It is as if the windows and doors appear open, but the normal internal responses have been turned well down. Sometimes people express this look by saying that the Metal type looks 'empty'.

THE EMOTIONAL CAPACITY OF THE METAL ELEMENT

The Metal Element gives us certain capacities. We can describe them as:

♦ The ability to feel loss and move on.
♦ The capacity to take in quality or richness from the outside world in order to feel complete.

So how does this ability relate to the Lungs? Chinese medicine tells us that the Lungs take in Qi from the Heavens. 'Qi' and 'Heaven' require some explanation.

Qi and Heaven

'Qi' can be described as our 'vital energy'. We can't normally see Qi but it gives us the ability to move, have vitality, keep warm and protect ourselves against disease. Without Qi running through our bodies we wouldn't be alive. The vital spark would be lost. The Chinese described the 'Heavens' as 'the highest cosmic principle or force' and 'the force which governs all of nature'.

Receiving Richness and Quality

If we have a healthy Metal Element and strong Lungs we can receive this cosmic energy from the heavens. This allows us to feel that we have richness and quality in our lives and that we are substantial human beings. Curiously, this sense of richness and quality is probably taken for granted by non-Metal types — like fish not noticing the water. Metal types, on the other hand, will experience it as fluctuating or absent.

This 'receiving of quality' manifests in many small ways. Acknowledgement from the people around us enables us to feel worthwhile. When we are young, people respond to us in various ways. Their positive responses help us to form our sense of self-worth. Our mothers pick us up, feed us and talk to us. Our parents guide us in various ways. Others who are older and wiser, such as teachers, aunts, uncles and grandparents, may give us recognition.

Receiving Acknowledgement and Recognition

The response or acknowledgement we get from the world contributes to our feeling of richness and quality. Sometimes a response is neutral; someone is simply aware of us. But often recognition is tinged with approval or disapproval. For example, some 'good' responses might be ones of gratitude, appreciation, thankfulness, honours, awards, credit or rewards. On the other hand, some 'bad' responses might be ones of disapproval, censure, rejection, discredit, condemnation, punishment or blame.

Positive acknowledgement helps us to learn that we are special and worthwhile human beings. It also leads, in normal circumstances, to an experience of satisfaction — that elusive state that so many of us are searching to find. The issue for the Metal type is the impaired ability to take in recognition.

EMOTIONS WE EXPERIENCE WHEN THE ABILITY IS IMPAIRED

Typically, the distinguishing emotional states of a Metal type are:

♦ Bereft, grief-stricken, incomplete or inadequate
♦ Not recognized or misunderstood.

Bereft, Grief-Stricken, Incomplete or Inadequate

A natural and appropriate feeling of grief or loss is stimulated if we suffer a loss in our life. When someone close dies, we feel, for a period of time, bereft. We miss the person and wish they were still with us. Over time we heal and this emotion disperses. Depending upon the closeness and our general strength, the time to disperse will vary.

Metal types have feelings generated in this way, but the *underlying* feeling of being bereft or incomplete feels similar in tone, but different because it has no associated loss. It is as if a loss has occurred, but with nothing actually missing. This can lead to a confusion. Charles described this:

> We were driving off to a picnic once and I had this nagging voice inside saying something wasn't quite right. It wasn't. We had forgotten the picnic hamper. But the way I feel a lot of the time is that there is something missing, but it isn't a picnic hamper or anything I can ever put my finger on. It's strange.

This feeling of loss comes from not being able to receive Qi from the heavens. It can be compared to a handful of earth which lacks vital minerals and trace elements which is wondering what is wrong with itself. Metal types may continuously feel that something is absent from their lives but may be unable to pinpoint what it is. Mark told us:

> I think grief is something I settle into. It's like an emptiness, there's nothing there to be grieving about. My mother used to say, 'you look really sad sometimes'. She noticed it in my expression. I think about what my life could have been like — when I'm really down that goes through my mind a lot.

Other Metal types feel a sense of grief about events or special times in their lives. Marion said:

> I often have a sense of having lost something. I feel as if I had something and it's now missing. Sometimes something really simple happens and I think, 'Oh I've not got that any more.' With my children I wish I could go back to the time they were little or I want to go back to other precious times. I think this leads me to be in the moment more acutely than someone else, so it adds pleasure, but it's still tinged with sadness.

When Metal types lament the past they might use words such as, 'If only such and such had happened, but it didn't ...' The accompanying feelings are sadness, regret, emptiness, loss.

Tears are a normal expression of grief, but Metal types are often private and have difficulty crying. The impulse may be there, but the energy of the chest is weak or blocked. The Metal type may worry that these feelings will overwhelm them and that the recognition by others would be invasive. Frederick describes:

I once cried at a party and I couldn't stand peoples' responses. They all tried to be nice and ask if I was all right, but they felt like vultures. It is much easier to deny the feelings.

Belinda's description is similar:

I never cry in public and I wouldn't like others to know I was upset. I often go through phases where I feel like crying a lot. If I do cry I'll only do it on my own.

BEREAVEMENT AND OUR IMMUNE SYSTEM

The immune systems of people who have recently been bereaved can become severely suppressed. This can leave them open to infections and many other illnesses. In 1975, twenty-six bereaved spouses took part in a study along with another twenty-six people who acted as a control group. Those who were bereaved were tested two weeks after the bereavement and again six weeks later. The immune systems of those who had lost a loved one were seriously suppressed, whilst those of the control group remained normal.[2]

Not Recognized or Misunderstood

The pattern of finding it hard to take in acknowledgement can leave a Metal type feeling dissatisfied, emotionally isolated and misunderstood. These feelings can intensify the search for meaning or for a connection to something outside themselves. Joan described it in this way:

Receiving is quite difficult. It's hard to believe that someone means something positive. I find it hard to be open to someone else in terms of receiving. It leaves me feeling too fragile and then I feel alone.

Recognition is so important for Metal types that it has to be totally sincere in order for them to take it in. Any hint of superficiality can mean that the complement is discarded. Marion, who we spoke to earlier, explained:

> It's difficult to hear good things about me. Something has to be said carefully in order for me to take it in and I listen very carefully. An insincere compliment is irritating. Something genuine, if their heart is in it, means a lot even if it is only a small thing and I treasure it deeply.

For Dennis the acknowledgement is never deep enough:

> When others give recognition, it feels insignificant and that somehow the other person doesn't see who I really am.

Flippancy is definitely not appreciated when it comes to meaningful issues. A Metal type feels deeply and takes life seriously.

LOSS AND DIABETES

A study carried out in Sweden in 1991 found that the loss of a family member could increase the risk of children succumbing to juvenile onset diabetes. If a child between the ages of 5 and 9 years had an actual loss *or was even threatened with a loss* this significantly increased the risk of the young person getting the disease.[3]

Recognizing the Emotion of a Metal Type in Everyday Life

We know that Metal types have difficulty receiving quality and richness from the outside world. This can make it hard for them to take in recognition from others if they have done something well.

In everyday life it is important to notice the kind of compliment or recognition being given. One level of respect is reflected by, 'Wow, you look good today!' A somewhat deeper level of respect is reflected by, 'You were very generous and very sensitive to that person — you have a special quality of kindness.' The latter kind would be more difficult for the Metal type to take in.

We might observe a Metal type receiving a compliment. They may deny that the recognition is deserved — by saying that anyone could have done it or that the accomplishment was really a trivial one. This is pushing away or denial. For this reason Metal types are often hard to praise.

Another response is a kind of deadness or simply a lack of response. It is obvious that they are not going to take the 'gift' in. If we look closer, however, we may notice a tightening up in the chest, a choking in the throat and possibly a welling up of tears. The beginnings of taking in are there, but the process has been interrupted.

Metal types may also avoid the expression of grief. The father of a friend of ours recently died. His wife who is an Earth type commented that she didn't think he had truly grieved over his death. 'He seemed to almost shrug it off,' she said, 'but I'm sure the feelings are still locked up somewhere inside him.' The Metal type will tend to shy away from emotional expressions of grief.

These are the kinds of observations you can make in everyday life and they may help to confirm that you are with a Metal type. So, how can we express what is important to the Metal type?

BIG ISSUES AND UNANSWERED QUESTIONS FOR THE METAL TYPE

For any type, when typical negative experiences recur, certain issues become more important than any others. The Big Issues for the Metal type are:

♦ Recognition
♦ Feeling complete
♦ Feeling adequate in the world
♦ Finding meaningfulness

To say that these are Big Issues is to say that in any situation, particularly one of stress, the Metal type will be concerned with whether they have been recognized, whether their imperfections are obvious and to whom, whether they are adequate to the situation, whether they are doing something meaningful. Depending on the strategies the Metal type has chosen, some of these will be more important than others.

Another way of expressing the internal experience of someone whose Metal is constitutionally impaired is that they begin, to varying degrees, to carry certain unanswered questions:

♦ Am I *really* OK, not specifically, but just generally OK?
♦ What is missing?
♦ What do I need to be complete?
♦ How can I truly connect with the world and therefore be complete?
♦ What will give my life meaning?

For the non-Metal type, there are answers to these questions. For the Metal type, these questions come up again and again, and to varying degrees do not get answered. The difficulty in finding answers to these questions can lead a Metal type to develop various life-patterns or strategies.

HOW WOULD YOU KNOW THAT YOUR FRIEND IS A METAL TYPE?

He or she might:
♦ Look bright white by and/or under the eyes
♦ Have a voice which tails off at the end of sentences
♦ Look slightly caved in in the chest
♦ Often seem to keep themselves aloof; although present, may seem distant
♦ Keep her or himself very active
♦ Seem very concerned about the purpose or meaning of what they do
♦ Seem to want recognition but be unable to take it in

RESPONSES TO THE BIG ISSUES

The ways of coping which we will discuss next are a response to the Big Issues and Unanswered Questions. Given that these issues are important and that the questions keep recurring, these are the kinds of lifestyles or behaviours which a Metal type might adopt to deal with their issues.

Not every Metal type will use all of these strategies and there may be other variations which we haven't observed. It is also possible for other types to behave in similar ways. In this case the behaviours might be less pronounced or have a different set of questions behind them.

The responses are:

♦ Distancing and protecting
♦ Doing well and doing more

♦ Resignation and cynicism
♦ Seeking quality
♦ Relating to the Father

Distancing and Protecting

Metal types are frequently described as distant or, in the extreme, 'cut off'. This may manifest as a reserve in the presence of others or simply hiding away in one's room. It can also manifest as working more in one's head, for example, as an academic.

People can distance themselves by working through social roles where closeness and personal exposure are kept to a minimum. Without doubt, most Metal types do not 'blab on' about their genuine personal concerns. This may be true of all types to some degree, but more so with Metal types. Here Dennis, who spoke earlier, explains his reasons keeping distant:

> Others don't always see who I am, so I don't get recognition. Things that are the most precious and valuable I have kept to myself and revealed only cautiously and only in the most trustworthy circumstances. I'm loathe to do it in a public way. I think it's the fear of the consequences of being misunderstood.

Distancing occurs for several reasons. Chinese medicine teaches that the skin is the body-part associated with the Metal Element. When the Lungs are weak the Metal type can feel very 'thin-skinned' and delicate.

This emotional fragility is also connected with a weakened P'o which is the mental-spiritual aspect of the Lungs. Earlier we discussed how the P'o protects us from unwanted mental or psychic influences. Physically we are protected by the Lung's defensive Qi and psychically by the P'o. When our Lungs are weak we are more vulnerable to those influences. Distancing compensates for our feelings of being fragile and enables the Metal type to appear to be all right to the outside world, even when they are feeling terrible inside. Marion explains this:

> Letting things show is messy, out of control and awkward. It really shows up my vulnerability. I'm tremendously fragile underneath and will only share it occasionally. On the surface I have to appear OK. The way I look and the things around me have to create harmony. I won't let any volatile emotions show through. It's best for me if everything is OK. If not, it's best to make it look OK and cope rather than fall apart.

Frequently Metal types will be very careful about which part of themselves is exposed — for fear, perhaps, that the sense of incompleteness or emptiness will be seen by others who might be critical. Belinda tells us:

I withdraw for self-defence. Especially if I feel a failure or I'm lacking in confidence. I don't show it to others, in fact I come over to others as very arrogant sometimes. It's important not to show that to others as I feel very fragile in my sense of self. I'm very vulnerable to what others say and do. I cut myself off and don't let others in. It makes me feel very alone at times.

We called the pattern 'distancing and protecting'. From the outside, it appears as distancing; from inside, it is experienced as protecting. Another way of coping can be to work hard.

Doing Well and Doing More

Metal types may have difficulty receiving quality or richness in their lives. This can lead them to feel incomplete. To compensate for this feeling, Metal types may try to bring quality into their lives through doing things exceptionally well. Alternatively, they might make up for it with quantity instead of quality. In this case they might work very hard.

It may not be possible to be good at everything, so often a Metal type will try to be outstanding in one specific area. Whatever the Metal type attempts to do in life, they will do so with effort aimed at doing well. Dennis tells us:

The word perfection comes to mind. I've always been like it from the moment I started reading and writing. Everything I've ever done has to be the best — it's almost obsessive — I'm beginning to tackle it, it's a big theme. When I decide to do something I put myself into it completely. The state of ambivalence is not for me — I find it extremely uncomfortable.

The task that is done may be being a mother and housewife, a nuclear physicist or solving crossword puzzles. The theme that runs through all of these is the Metal type's motivation to do it well. As 'doing well' is usually hard to define, this leaves the Metal type open to criticism that what has been done is not really as good as it might be — it could have been just that little bit better. These criticisms can come from others but frequently from Metal types themselves. One Metal type described this process:

It is setting impossible standards for the world around me so I am easily disappointed by people who do not live up to those standards, but equally I can disappoint myself because my standards are impossible for *me* to obtain — I am left constantly striving and constantly wanting to do things better and better and better.

This constant internal criticism means that the Metal type will be short on satisfaction. Satisfaction is often the result of positive acknowledgement, so one of the theme songs for a Metal type could be 'I can't get no satisfaction'.

'Satisfaction' is that emotional and physically-felt state of pleasure which is associated with having done something well. Satisfaction can be gained from having typed 20 letters, or given a speech, or enrolled a child in a nursery, or helped a neighbour. It is a natural and nourishing event.

Metal types who use this strategy will lack this final sense of accomplishment. Often when they reach the moment for satisfaction at the end of a job well done they simply cannot or do not take it in. They may sabotage their results or simply move on to something else knowing quite well that they could be doing just that little bit better. As Dennis put it:

There's no time for sitting around just feeling good when you could be doing more and getting closer to perfection.

A variation on 'doing well' is doing something better than others and using the external performance to generate massive amounts of attention and acknowledgement. It is as if Metal types know they have difficulty taking in the rewards so they make the rewards or acknowledgement enormous. They act as if more will be better, but it never is.

The Metal type might excel at almost anything — as long as it generates attention and acknowledgement. It could be making money. Money buys bigger cars, foreign villas, valuable jewellery or expensive schools for the children. Or it could be getting into the *Guinness Book of Records* or being the 'best' or simply 'very good' at something.

The question Metal types might ask themselves is: 'Does this activity of being excellent at something just generate attention and look good or does it give me internal satisfaction?' More on the outside does not mean more on the inside. So the quandary remains the same — taking in the attention is the issue, not generating massive amounts of it.

One of the consequences of feeling incomplete can be constant effort to do well. On the other hand, with very little effort, the Metal type can lapse into resignation.

Resignation and Cynicism

Metal types may give up inside because they know that whatever they do, it will never seem to be quite enough. There will always be something missing. This may be based on the experience of having tried many things and never found fulfilment. Teresa, a Metal type said:

> There is an emptiness in me all the time and this feeling that there is something better round the corner. In the end I always feel that, I come back to the same sort of emptiness. I feel like I am still where I was ten years ago.

One Metal type we know, whose name is Adam, got the nickname 'I-don't-give-a-damn-Adam'. This resulted from his frequently saying, when confronted by any even potential loss or disappointment that he 'did not give a damn'. James, another Metal type did something similar. He told us:

> I often feel misunderstood and then I say, 'Who gives a shit?' This is my way of dealing with feeling bad.

Resignation as a strategy could be described as a denial or avoidance of disappointment. If we have no stake in anything, there is nothing to lose.

A consequence which often accompanies resignation is a form of cynicism and a tendency to criticize. The effect of the belief that we are flawed has been taken by some Metal types to mean that their own efforts are worthless. It is a short step, and probably an inevitable one, to project that onto others. Their efforts to become special, to 'do well' and find meaning are ultimately foolish and doomed to failure too. For example Marion said:

> I can come away from situations feeling very disdainful and judgmental of other people sometimes and think, 'That was a waste of time,' even though they might be trying really hard. I'm critical of others as well as myself. I set impossible standards no one can reach.

A Metal type may be searching to find meaning and connection in a different way which we will talk about next.

Seeking Quality

Knowing that we are imperfect can lead a Metal type to formally or informally become a 'seeker'. This is really a searching for the quality and connection which they feel is missing from their life. It may manifest as seeking the ultimate connection which is with the spirit. Dennis put it this way:

> There are lots of things people find fun, but I often wonder why they are bothered — it's not that there is anything wrong with them, but you are going to die and the most important thing is spiritual, so it is finding a spiritual path and following that is important to me. It is a preoccupation with getting to what is really real. I feel really good when I connect, and that is not a connection with people.

The seeking may be carried out via a religious avenue where the satisfactions of material life are renounced and vows taken. It may, however, simply be done by a constant searching for quality or meaning through seeking knowledge, truth, beauty, the right organization to join, the right beliefs to adhere to or finding the right exercises or spiritual practice to follow. The need for perfection or completion is a driving force in the choices of life. Marion notices she seeks quality in many ways. One of these ways is by the clothes she wears:

> I buy the best clothes, I'm ridiculous, the ones I have must have a decent label. I will search for days looking for the right accessory.

She then went on to say:

> Quality in people is also important. They don't have to be intelligent but they do have to be genuine. I would be disappointed if they let me down or humiliated me — which I fear. Then cracks would appear.

Some Metal types, as a result of seeking, have been told that they are always changing — jobs, profession, spiritual practices or friends. They may appear to chop and change what they do and give the impression that their life is very erratic. At the heart of this may be a common thread as Dennis told us:

My quest appears to be inconsistent but in my experience it's been the same thing all along. It's the same project and it changes — it's all the quest for truth. I'm passionate about the truth.

Relating to the Father

This is not so much a strategy as an observed association. Metal types often relate strongly to the father in the family. They may have lost their father early and were unable to fully grieve as Jean told us:

> I think all my life I've had this feeling that I've lost something. I've never been able to put my finger on it. I think I first focused on it when my father died and it's something I've still never got over. It's an overwhelming sense of loss.

Metal types may have a very strong bond with their father which may be fondly recalled later in life or there may have been a lack of closeness. It is not the good or bad nature of the relationship but the importance of the father. Marion recalls:

> My own father was extraordinary. He left school at 11 and was self-educated. He ended up running a psychiatric hospital. I regretted my lack of closeness. Since my mother died we learnt to appreciate each other and I'm so grateful. I speak to him on the phone every day. I've lost my mother but I've gained something through it, but when I speak to him it's always tinged with the loss of my mother.

The relationship with the father may have to do with seeking what is perfect. Often, from the viewpoint of a child, the father is the ultimate authority and arbiter of right and wrong. Belinda told us:

> My father was always a problem for me. He was a huge influence on my life. He gave me compliments in front of people but never said anything nice to me when I was on my own with him. He always showed off about me and that was why I developed the way I did. I now tend to turn people into father figures. I put people up on pedestals as father figures. It's taken a long time to see people as human and I've given some people far too much respect.

There is a basis for the connection with the father in the theory of Chinese medicine. The Heavens represent the father and the Earth represents the mother.

People are often represented as standing being between Heaven and Earth. We need to be in contact with both. We can nourish ourselves with food from the Earth but still be lacking something because we have lost contact with the father.

The traditional Christian prayers have always been made to 'Our Father who art in Heaven' — although this has changed in the nineties, it is a tradition steeped in meaning. The Lungs, which receive the Qi energy from the heavens, are the main contact with the higher part of ourselves.

The Earth satisfies our more basic needs, but the Heavens are the location of our mental and spiritual nourishment. It is for this reason that many meditation exercises concentrate on our breathing. For heavenly inspiration, we do not look to the Earth. We look upwards to the Heavens.

Some Metal types seek a connection with an image of the father or something powerful outside themselves. This may be expressed through the spiritual search which we mentioned earlier, or by finding teachers or other 'father figures' to guide them. Alternatively, they may strive to prove to themselves that they are at least as strong and powerful as any father figure. One way of achieving this is by doing things such as endurance exercises, weight training or martial arts. Another way is to show that they can be totally independent and can cope without other people's help.

Metal types may have a conflict between becoming independent from a father figure and at the same time wanting more dependence and unity. Independence temporarily makes them feel more whole. They don't have to rely on anyone else — but they are isolated. Dependence temporarily gives them a feeling of being connected — but they can't always rely on that person to be there. In the end the Metal type may discover that the ultimate connection to the father or the cosmic force is not in the outside world, but in connecting to their own spiritual nature and realizing that they are already whole, complete and perfect.

VIRTUES AND VICES OF A METAL TYPE

Depending on the health of the Metal type, these ways of coping produce both virtues and vices. Some of the virtues are:

♦ Hard work
♦ Competence and often a high level of expertise
♦ Looking for the best and towards the best
♦ A degree of objectivity
♦ A useful longing for a connection with higher meaning.

> Some of the vices or imperfections are:
> ◆ Cutting off and becoming isolated
> ◆ Over-criticism of themselves or others
> ◆ An obsession with struggle and performance
> ◆ A cynical resignation
> ◆ An obsession with matters 'spiritual' to the detriment of those of
>   ordinary life.

A FAMOUS METAL TYPE — RICHARD FEYNMAN[4]

Metal type Richard Feynman is probably one of the most famous physicists of our time. He lived and worked in the United States and was well-known for his books, his service for the Challenger commission and for his numerous appearances on television. Beneath an outwardly friendly exterior was, however, a very serious man.

Metal types often like to be outstanding in one particular area of their lives and Feynman certainly knew how to be 'the best'. He strove for perfection in his work as a physicist. Many of his colleagues said he was a genius and certainly when he died in 1988 a book of reminiscences described him as 'brilliant', 'creative' and 'the most inventive of his generation'. It has been said that it is hard to name another scientist who commanded as much admiration and respect as he did — some even said he was greater than Einstein.

It is interesting to note how Feynman had a combination of some of the typical strategies found in many Metal types. Besides doing things well to the extent that he was called a genius, he also distanced himself from others. A colleague commented that no one ever got close to him and we might wonder if he could truly take in just how much he was admired. He was also unable to deal with the grief of losing his wife at an early age.

Feynman has also been described as 'the most independent cuss ever to walk the Earth'. He never took anyone else's word for anything. He loved to solve the problems of the universe. Being a scientist gave him the ability to understand those problems in a new and better way than anyone else and, what's more, in *his* way. He received a Nobel prize in 1965 for his work on the quantum theory of the electromagnetic field — described as one of the shining jewels of modern science.

Like many Metal types Richard Feynman had high standards for himself but could also be critical in the extreme. Visiting scientists often came to lecture at the Californian Institute of Technology where he worked. He would then invariably sit in the centre front row and taunt and hector anyone who didn't measure up to his high standards. He was a mixture of someone who strove to produce work of the highest quality and at the same time was cut off and isolated from many people.

As we mentioned earlier, Feynman never resolved his grief about the sad and early death of his first wife. How he dealt with this is a strange contradiction — although not so strange in the light of him being a Metal type. At the time of her death he said it left him 'curiously unmoved' and he then refused to let anyone comfort him after the funeral. Only three days after her death he rang a friend suggesting that they 'go and pick up a few girls'.

This contrasts with the fact that at the end of his life and forty years after her death he still wept uncontrollably for her. Two years after her death he wrote a letter to her which was filled with his heartbreak, loneliness and grief. This he preserved with some of her belongings in an ancient suitcase which he would occasionally bring out and gaze at with deep emotion.

He finally died of cancer in 1988 but he kept on working until the very end of his life. When asked how much he worked he said that he couldn't tell. He never knew when he was working or when he was playing.

GOLDEN RULES FOR METAL TYPES

♦ Find out how you are already deep-down perfect.
♦ Protect yourself and reach out to others.
♦ If only slowly, determine to let others know who you are, and check their understanding.
♦ As an experiment, assume things are easy.
♦ The 'forever' part of you is divine — spend time with it.

Notes

1   See Weiger, L, 1965: *Chinese Characters*; page 49.
2   'Depressed Lymphocyte Function after Bereavement', by RW Bartrop, L Lazarus, E Luckhurst, CG Kiloh and R Penny. Published in the *Lancet*, April 16 1977, pages 834–7.
3   'Stress and Metastasis', by Bruce McEwen and Elliot Stellar. Published by the *Archives of Internal Medicine*, September 27 1993, page 2097.
4   The information on Richard Fenyman is taken from Grenstein, George *'Portraits of Discovery'*, 1998.

Chapter 9

EXERCISES FOR METAL TYPES

INTRODUCTION

The exercises in this section are aimed at enabling Metal types to find a better emotional balance. Some useful goals for Metal types are:

- To recognize and take in positive acknowledgement
- To be aware of what drives them and, if appropriate, to soften the effect of their attempts to do well and more
- To convert cynicism into compassion
- To be open with others via objectivity and compassion
- To deal with their natural distancing which they use to protect themselves.

USING THE EXERCISES

We suggest that you read an exercise through before you start it. All of the exercises are laid out in a similar style. Following the *introduction*, we tell you approximately *how long* it will take to complete. Obviously some of you will take more time and others less. The exercises are then divided into stages. They start with:

- the *purpose* of the exercise and then
- the *process* or the steps of the exercise.

The theme of each step is in bold so that you have a summary. At the end of some exercises we have a section called *'matters arising'*. Here we discuss issues which could come up while you do the exercise.

THE EXERCISES FOR METAL TYPES

♦ Giving gifts
♦ Receiving gifts
♦ Educating others
♦ Checking out my standards
♦ Dealing with loss
♦ A Qigong exercise for moving energy through the chest
♦ A Qigong exercise for breathing fully

EXERCISE 1 — GIVING GIFTS

Introduction

David read this exercise and shook his head. He couldn't see the point of 'giving gifts', especially as, he said, he might not be able to do it sincerely. We reminded him that this exercise was a preparation for the next exercise and that maybe he could do this one and then find out more about 'why' when he did the second exercise. He said, 'All right', and completed the exercise. He said it *was* interesting watching people receive the 'gifts' and he was also surprised at how the 'gifts' affected people. He said he was looking forward to the second exercise, 'Receiving Gifts'.

Time required: 10 minutes preparation and half a minute at various times during the day.

Purpose

This exercise enables a Metal type to formulate compliments and observe several people receiving them. Its purpose is to familiarize us, from an observer's point of view, with what the process is like. It also anticipates the next exercise when we are on the receiving end of the 'gifts'. In addition, many people find the ability to give 'gifts' a valuable one.

Process

1 **Think of something you might say to another person which would be a compliment or indicate your respect for them.** Think of people you see regularly — people from your family, work, the shop, the post office, the pub or

wherever. This might seem new to you at first. So take a little time and write the things down that you might say. You know what a compliment is, but the best would be:

♦ Ones that arise from information you have about the person

♦ Ones that refer to something that would be important to them

♦ Ones which possibly refer to an internal quality they have rather than a physical one — although variety is fine.

Think about the best way to phrase what you are going to say to this person. You may even want to run through giving the compliment to the other person in your imagination to check if you have a good one.

2 **When you next see the person, give them the compliment.** It is like a free gift with no strings attached. You may have to be a bit ingenious and pick the best moment to give it. Give at least three compliments a day. It is even better to give five. Keep a notebook and record what happens.

3 **In the few seconds after making the gift, watch how the person takes it in.** Do they take it in:

♦ Smoothly

♦ Have a good feeling in their chest

♦ Say, 'Thank you', or acknowledge what you said in some way?

Remember that you are noticing how they take the compliment in. Get to the stage that you can decide on the degree to which someone 'received' the compliment. For example, so you can discriminate:

♦ Someone for whom it was really easy,

♦ Someone who found it difficult but could do it, and

♦ Someone who avoided or rejected it.

Do this for at least a week and record your observations in your notebook.

4 **Speculate about the consequences of your gifts.** Write your speculations down in your notebook. Did people benefit? How? For those who took the compliments in, specific questions might be:

♦ Might they have had a better day?

♦ Could you have changed their view of themselves at all?

♦ Will their relationships with others improve?

♦ If a lot of people did this regularly, what might happen?

EXERCISE 2 — RECEIVING GIFTS

Introduction

David, from Exercise 1, approached this exercise with some interest. Something had touched him when watching people receive gifts. He said he knew instinctively that receiving 'gifts' was an emotional issue for him. He said, 'I think I have some strong feelings about doing this.' This turned out to be true. At first it was difficult for him to find 'internal' compliments. He said he was determined to succeed and he did take more time to complete step 5. He said, however, that he now understood what had fascinated him when watching others receive gifts and that he had learned some very important things about himself. Steps 6–8 were also fascinating and after three weeks he said that the exercise seemed to be changing him in quite a deep way.

Time needed: 15–30 minutes.

Purpose

This exercise is designed to develop your capacity to take in good feelings, compliments and respect in such a way that it nourishes you.[1] For this exercise it is particularly useful to ask someone else to read the process and direct you. The help of another person increases your chances enormously of getting definite benefits.

Process

1 Write down at least ten:
   ♦ Good feelings you could have about yourself
   ♦ Compliments you could pay yourself, or
   ♦ Things you could say to yourself demonstrating how you feel respect for yourself.

   Metal types are often a little slower than others at this task so make sure you take some time.

   The things you write down may be physical:
   ♦ You look attractive when you dress well.
   ♦ Twenty press-ups is a lot considering you could not do 5 a month ago ...
   Or they may be to do with your capacities:

♦ You accomplish a lot at work when you put your mind to it.

♦ You have a way of knowing what's going to happen that is special.

♦ You understand Alan better than anyone I know.

Or they may be — and these àre preferable — internal, maybe moral qualities:

♦ You are good with your partner — even though she is difficult you are always fair and decent.

♦ After watching you with X, Y and Z, I have to say that you are very kind and generous.

♦ You have a seriousness and determination which means the company never can forget its purpose.

Whatever you do, keep what you say simple and leave out any qualifications. Also, make sure you get the words just right. For example, one of these may be better than the other:

♦ I like the way you dealt with Sandra. It wasn't easy for you and yet you were understanding and compassionate towards her.

♦ You were great with Sandra, really kind, really compassionate and very understanding.

Some of you may not be able to find anything of this sort to say to yourself. That's fine. You could write down — as a compliment — that you are not one to take in flattery easily! You could also try harder. You could also use the alternative approach written below.

2 **Start thinking of the things that someone else might or does appreciate about you.** As before, these can be good feelings, compliments or things that could be respected about you. Some people are always going around saying nice things to others — be like one of them. If you need to make these appreciations tiny or just trivial little things, that's all right too. Write ten of them down. It doesn't matter if *you* don't think they are true or worthwhile. Just put them into the words that would sound best to you — if others were to appreciate you.

3 **Now, take one of these ten and say it out loud to yourself.** It might be useful to use two chairs. Sit in one chair and put an image of yourself in the other. If your name is Steve and the compliment is that you have really done a good job on project X, then say out loud:

♦ Steve (your name), you really have done a good job on project X.

Change to the chair opposite and notice how you respond both in your mind and in your body. For example, you might in your mind be saying: 'Actually I could have done a better job,' or 'It was easy — never even stretched me,' or 'Who are you to tell me — you don't know how hard I worked,' and so on. In your body, you might be pulling back a bit, tightening your chest, looking away, sensing a barrier of feelings between you and the 'you' who is delivering the message.

You may also be saying, 'Yes, I did do a good job,' and feeling just a little pleased with being acknowledged — even though it is you doing the acknowledging and this *is* just an exercise.

As you do this, write down what you are thinking and feeling in response to what you have said.

4 **Take the other things you might say to yourself one by one** and repeat what you did in step 3. Collect more information about what you do when you receive positive information about yourself. Repeat this up to ten times, continuing to write down what comes up in your mind and in your body.

5 **Read through what you have written down and ask yourself, 'What stops me from taking acknowledgement, compliments and good feelings about myself?'** Write down any answers you get. The kind of responses that people record are: 'I tighten my throat and chest so no feeling can pass,' or 'I don't trust what people say; they don't really know,' but you decide how you do it.

6 **Now, use the same statements, and where necessary changing your words and voice tone. Find a way of receiving them even if it is in a limited or small way.**

7 **Write down the feelings and thoughts you have** as you do take the compliments in. Notice what it is like taking them in rather than keeping them out.

8 **Work on this exercise every day.** Take at least five good things to say to yourself. Your goal is to take them in in the following way:

♦ With a smooth flow of feeling
♦ Having a good feeling somewhere in the chest area
♦ With a fluent response where you acknowledge the compliment or respect and say, 'Thank you'. Taking the last example you might say to yourself, 'Thank you Steve, yes I did do a good job.'

As you practise this exercise over a period of time, notice how your response to acknowledgement or compliments changes.

EXERCISE 3 — EDUCATING OTHERS

Introduction

Eddie spent a lot of time grouching. He worked as part of a team and always wanted to be included. On the other hand, he seemed endlessly to complain about how the team functioned. The other team members, who liked and appreciated him, never quite knew what was wrong. Eddie did this exercise and after three weeks, in a meeting, one of his colleagues mentioned how positive he had been. Eddie, as part of the exercise, had been doing some 'educating' and realized that others did not know what he'd been doing. After two months, he described the exercise as 'Ace', which in his language meant it was special.

Time needed: 2–3 minutes a few times a day.

Purpose

This exercise is designed to help Metal types to understand why they need to distance themselves. At the same time it gives them the flexibility to find ways to gain protection and be treated well. A Metal type may be reluctant to reveal their hurt feelings or needs. Learning how to educate other people's behaviour in the right direction leads to greater satisfaction and a feeling of being more in control.

Process

1 **Think of five situations when people behaved insensitively towards you and caused you to feel hurt or offended.** You may have brushed these incidents off as 'not important', or even said you didn't care, but they can be large or very, very small. Jot down a word or two to remind yourself of each.
2 **For each, write down:** What the other person did not know about you and how you would like them to approach you in the future.

These could be as simple as:

♦ They don't know that I hate to be interrupted when I am working at my computer.
♦ I would like them to ask me if I am willing to talk about a certain subject, rather than assuming it and just launching in and talking.

The issues can be small or large.

3 **Imagine responding to each person with a request that they change their behaviour.** Consider what you might say. You may find the following format useful:
    ♦ Identify the relevant event: *'You know when you ...'*
    ♦ Say exactly how you are sensitive: *'I do not like ...'*
    ♦ Explain it as rationally as you can — you can even say you don't understand why you feel the way you do.
    ♦ Say how you would like them to behave differently, *'I would appreciate it if instead you ...'*
    Alternatively, using the same example, you could use a more indirect approach where you simply say out of the blue and without reference to any previous incident:

    You know what I really, really appreciate? I'm deep in thought and somebody comes up to talk, but first they ask me if I am willing. I think that's really great when somebody does that. It shows real thoughtfulness.

    (Remember Exercise 1, 'Giving Gifts' and make this a potential gift.)
4 **Ask yourself whether you could actually make the five 'requests'.** What would happen? How would you feel? Would it be dangerous?
    Consider two alternatives. One is that no one knows what you expect and people will often approach you in ways you find offensive. The other is that if people knew how you like to be treated they would be more considerate.
    Ask yourself whether it would be worth educating a few people to be more sensitive to you. This may be especially important for people who are significant in your life.
5 **Communicate with four to five people per week telling them how you like to be treated.** Remember you are making a request and at the same time making your needs known. Assume that this is a long-term strategy. Lots of people will forget what you said or simply not understand it. Assume a low rate of immediate successes, but think about the cumulative effect of even occasional successes.
6 **Over a few months, notice how your new habit is progressing.** Notice what its consequences are. People may be behaving differently. You could find yourself being much clearer about what you would like to receive from other people. The amount of misunderstanding or hurt you experience could be reducing. Remember, you can always choose not to say anything. Whether you make a request or not is completely under your control.

Matters Arising

You may think, 'But I shouldn't have to ask people — that makes their behaviour worthless — they should just understand me.' Remember how each type is different. You may also wonder how much you know about what others want. Even if you do know sometimes, you do not *always* know.

EXERCISE 4 — CHECKING OUT MY STANDARDS

Introduction

Bill was someone who did most things to incredibly high standards. He was a clinical psychologist and his wife occasionally complained that he unnecessarily brought cases home to review and she and the children were neglected.

Bill was fond of saying, 'If you do something, do it well — or don't do it at all.' One day Bill's wife, with a very big smile, responded by saying, 'Absolutely, and that goes for being a husband and a father.' Bill was quiet and, without saying so, a little hurt, but he got the message. He used this exercise to look at the different areas of his life. The overall result was that he became more conscious of his various standards and made some adjustments in favour of his wife and kids.

Time needed: 15–20 minutes.

Purpose

This exercise is aimed at helping Metal types to consider what their standards are. It will also enable them to consider whose standards they are working to. Metal types often do too much or try to do better than other people. This is because they are trying to find meaning and quality in their lives. Considering the standards they are working to can give them a conscious chance to accept them or to change them.

Process

1 **List two to five areas where you are concerned about how well you do or where you push yourself to do too much.** These could include activities such as a relationship, work, going to the sports club, parenting, rally driving or racing pigeons. You may not have thought about these activities in this way before, so take your time to specify them.

2 **For each activity, one at a time, use three rating categories and write down as many of the criteria as you can for:**
   ♦ how you might do them well
   ♦ how they could be done satisfactorily, but not necessarily to the highest standards
   ♦ What would be not doing them well enough.

   It might help you if you take a sheet of paper. Draw columns down the page for the activities and three rows across for the rating categories. Enter your specific criteria in the boxes created.

	Relationship	Work	Sports Club	Parenting	Rally Driving
Done poorly					
Satisfactory					
Done well					

Figure 11: CHECKING OUT MY STANDARDS

3 **One activity at a time, examine your standards** and ask these questions.
   ♦ Are they accurate, for example, if you meet the 'doing well' standard, do you believe you have done well and do you acknowledge this?
   ♦ In the light of the 'Receiving Gifts' exercise above, when you meet the 'doing well' standard, do you take it in and feel some satisfaction? This is a crucial question.
   ♦ Are the standards reasonable or are they somehow all a little high?
   ♦ Are the standards negative ones (about what you *do not* want to happen) or are they positive (what you *do* want to happen)?
   ♦ Are the standards balanced, e.g. do you do some things too well and others less well?

EXERCISE 5 — DEALING WITH LOSS

Introduction

Jessie was Sally's dog and had been her 'best friend' throughout some very difficult teenage years. In spite of being old, Jessie would still greet her with enthusiasm and want to nuzzle her and be with her. When Jessie died Sally was grief stricken.

After five weeks of spontaneous weeping, Sally knew she was stuck in her feelings and neglecting other parts of her life. She asked her acupuncture practitioner to help and she was taken through the following exercise. At the end she said, 'I know it will be easier now. I don't think anyone else — even me — has understood what Jessie meant to me. But I do now and it's okay to let go and move on.'

Time needed: 15–25 minutes.

Purpose

This exercise is a process for dealing with loss. It can enable anyone who is stuck in the process of grieving to move on. It is natural to grieve when we lose someone close to us, but losses can also take many other forms. We can lose status, a dream we have about ourselves, a pet, a job, athletic or any other skills, a happy childhood or youthfulness. It is the *meaning* of what we lose which determines the extent of the loss.

This exercise can benefit any type but we have placed it with the exercises for Metal types as they often have the most difficulties with grief and loss.[2]

Process

1 **Think of either a loss which you can't let go of or a loss for which you feel you have never fully grieved.** The former will be an ongoing sore. Probably whenever you think of the loss you re-enter negative feelings. For the latter, you are probably more bothered by the lack of grieving than you are the loss. The former is better for this exercise.

2 **Remind yourself of the loss and notice how you think about it.** The loss doesn't have to be of a person. It can include a pet, a job, a dream or any of the examples given above. Find an image of what you have lost and note:

   ♦ The location of your image. Is it in front of you or to the left or right? Is it above eye-level or below? How far away is it?

   ♦ The quality of the image. Is it in colour or black and white, fuzzy or clear, bright or dark, moving or still, are you in the picture or not?

   ♦ Any sound in the image. If there are voices, what is their tone, where they are coming from and what is the volume and the tempo?

   ♦ This image will often be small, distant and not easily accessible to you.

3 **Now think of someone or something else which you have lost but which you feel fine about now.** It is not that the loss was not important, but

just that you have recovered from it. Notice the qualities of this image in the same way as in step 2. Note down:

♦ The location of your image. Is it in front of you or to the left or right? Is it above eye-level or below? How far away is it?

♦ What is the quality of the image: Is it in colour or black and white, fuzzy or clear, bright or dark, moving or still, are you in the picture or not?

♦ Any sound in the image. If there are voices, what is their tone, where they are coming from and what is the volume and the tempo?

You now know the difference between how your brain recognizes a loss which you are still grieving for and one which you have recovered from and which you feel fine about.

4 **Think of some of the pleasant things you remember about who or what you have lost.** Take a pleasant memory of the person, situation or event that you are grieving for. Move this image to the place in the second example which is reserved for when you have recovered from a loss.

First move the location of your image. Then change the other characteristics of the image so that it is of the same quality and has the same sounds as the second image. You can now expect to feel much more positive about the person, situation or event you were grieving for.

5 **Now review some of the good experiences you felt with the person, situation or event.** If it was a close friend you lost, these may include qualities or values such as, 'closeness', 'the ability to be myself', 'we had fun together', 'passion', or 'intimacy'.

6 **Take five of these qualities or values and form an image of them.** Do this in whatever way you want. This will often be a symbolic image such as light, brightness or sunshine. See yourself in the future, enjoying these qualities or values again in a fulfilling way in a new situation. Doing this will enable you to move on from your grief and take these satisfying qualities on into your future life.[3]

QIGONG EXERCISE FOR MOVING ENERGY THROUGH THE CHEST

Introduction

Nino is a Metal type. When doing a Qigong seminar, the teacher in passing told him to let his chest move more when he breathed. Nino already knew his chest did not move much and that it felt internally inert. This incident made him resolve to do something about it. He asked for and was given the following exercise. After two months of regular practice, he says that he notices more movement and occasionally he has a feeling of warmth for others which comes upwards from his lower abdomen and goes through his chest. He said he had never felt that before and has resolved to continue the exercise.

Time needed: 5–10 minutes daily.

Purpose

The purpose of this exercise is mentally to move energy through the area of the Lungs and thereby strengthen the capacity of the Lungs.

Process

1 **Stand with your feet shoulders' width apart and your knees slightly bent.** Keep the inside edges of your feet parallel. From your hips, bounce gently up and down an inch or so. Feel how your weight travels down from your hips to your feet which are solid on the floor. Tuck your tailbone in so that your lower back is straight. Notice any differences between each of your legs and any feelings of discomfort, heaviness or thickness. Allow your arms to hang by your sides with your palms turned slightly outwards so your armpits feel open. Draw your chin in slightly so that your spine stretches upward. Relax your chest and let the front of your abdomen drop.

2 **Rotate your hands.** Slowly rotate the right hand clockwise and the left anti-clockwise. End up with the palms facing each other and holding an imaginary ball in front of your groin. Now allow your fingers to drop slightly so that they point more directly towards your toes. This will allow the junction between your thumb and your wrist to open slightly.

3 **On a long in-breath, allow the hands and arms to move upwards.** Move the arms up until they are level with the ground and extended straight in front of you. As you do this imagine that a string is attached to a place at the junction between your thumb and wrist and that the string helps pull the arms up. You may also imagine or feel that the in-breath helps to move the arms up. After you learn the whole movement, you may feel, as the arms move up, that energy is moving up from your abdomen and through your chest.

4 Turn the palms to face the ground and on the out-breath allow the arms to move downwards to their original position. As the arms descend, feel the palms of your hands pressing down to the earth and feel energy moving out of the end of your fingers.

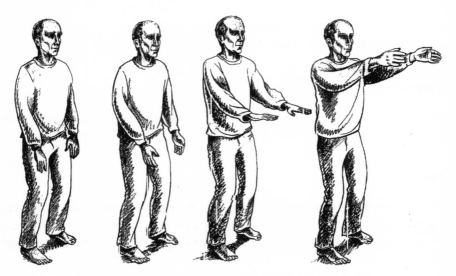

Figure 12: QIGONG EXERCISE FOR MOVING ENERGY THROUGH THE CHEST

Matters Arising

When learning this exercise, it can be easier to forget about the breath and any of the internal sensations. First practise turning the hands and moving the arms up and down. When you are ready, add the string pulling up at the wrist. Then look out for the internal upward movement through the abdomen and chest and feelings in the palms and fingers on the way down.

QIGONG EXERCISE FOR BREATHING FULLY

Introduction

After Penny discovered she was a Metal type, she noticed that she rarely breathed fully. She asked her practitioner for a breathing exercise and was given the following. After a month's practise, she says she feels larger throughout her abdomen and more relaxed in her shoulders. She does about 10 minutes a day and is anticipating more benefits.

Time required: 5–10 minutes daily.

Purpose

To direct attention to the breathing process and to enable it to become fuller. To increase energy flow from the lower to upper abdomen.

Process

1   You can do this exercise either standing, lying or sitting in a chair. If you do it standing **stand with your feet shoulder width apart and the inside edges of your feet parallel.** Allow your arms to hang by your sides with your palms turned slightly outwards so your armpits feel open. If you do it lying, **lie flat on your back on a flat surface without a cushion for your head.** Your legs should be straight. If you **sit in a chair,** sit near the front edge so your back is not supported and put your feet flat on the floor and shoulder width apart. The chair's seat should be high enough that the angle behind the knee and the angle between the upper part of the body and the thighs is at least 90 degrees.

2   **Place the palms of your hands on your lower abdomen** so that they can sense the lower abdomen's movement as you breathe in and out. Breathe in through your nose and out through your mouth. At first just notice the rising of your lower abdomen as the breath comes in and the lowering as the breath goes out. Later you can allow the out-breath to be longer and gently encourage the lower abdomen to rise more on the in-breath.

3   **After breathing this way for a time, move your hands up to your midriff or diaphragm** and lay them so the tips of your middle fingers are an inch or two apart. Continue to breathe as before, but allow the breath to expand you sideways. Notice how far an in-breath moves your fingers apart.

Wherever your hands are, simply pay attention to your breathing — as it comes in and as it goes out. Never strain. You should become more and more relaxed. Continue for 5 to 10 minutes.

Notes

1   This exercise was introduced to us by Marty Fromm who is a Gestalt therapist in Miami. We have used it in a variety of ways and thank Marty both personally and professionally.

2 Andreas, Connirae and Andreas, Steve, 1989: *Heart of the Mind*; Real People Press, Moab, Utah, pages 110—20.

3 The authors referred to in note 2 above also suggest using this process to pre-grieve. If a loss is forthcoming, e.g. a divorce is starting or a partner is dying, pre-grieving can help you to let go now. This does not mean that, for example, with a loved one who is dying, you actually let go of the relationship; it just means that access to those qualities/values and the good feelings associated with them does not have to be lost.

Chapter 10

THE WATER TYPE - REASSURING OURSELVES

FRANK IS A WATER TYPE

Frank is a Water type and is in his late forties. He is a barrister by profession. 'I chose to go into the bar partly because it would challenge me. I knew that if I could handle the bar I could overcome my fears. Being in adversarial situations where people are going for me, means my situation always feels slightly dangerous.'

Frank is highly sought after for his skilled approach to people. 'Because I'm so aware of how it is to feel afraid, I can create a space for people to express themselves. I'm told I bring a sense of calm to the situation. My alertness and slight wariness have in turn given me an ability to read people well.'

Frank is also valued for his sensitive strategies in dealing with his clients, 'I'm aware that I approach most situations with caution. I'm often thinking, "This could happen," or, "If this happens, how would I deal with it?" I tend to look at all of the angles and think "What if..." Which means I do my job thoroughly.

'People say that in my work I sometimes step in where angels fear to tread. I know I do, but I'm never reckless. It's more that I'm taking a calculated chance. For example, I recently had to steer a cross examination between a number of important areas. My assistant thought I was taking a high-risk strategy. I had enough confidence to know I could steer things through. It worked, thank goodness!'

Like many other Water types Frank has a blue hue to his face, especially by the eyes. He also has a slightly monotone sound to his voice. Along with his fear and caution these also indicate that he is a Water type.

As you read the rest of this chapter, you may understand more about Frank and why he is a Water type. We will begin by looking at the Water Element in Chinese medicine.

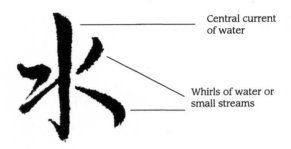

Central current of water

Whirls of water or small streams

Figure 13: THE CHINESE CHARACTER FOR WATER

THE WATER ELEMENT IN NATURE

The Chinese character for Water is 'shui' which is drawn above. This 'picture' represents a central current of Water with smaller streams flowing at either side. It depicts the flowing and moving nature of Water.[1]

Like water, our emotions flow. As such, they should flow smoothly, appearing, rising, falling and disappearing. Our emotions are like a river which can tumble over rocks, course through underground streams or pour through narrow gullies. Water is extremely soft and finds its way round many obstacles. Over time it can wear away the hardest rock and make it smooth. When we are balanced emotionally we also can 'flow' through our lives unhindered.

There are times, however, when a river does not flow smoothly. It can be frozen over or dammed up or burst its banks through flooding. The emotion fear, which is associated with the Water Element, clearly can block the flow of our energy. Fear often creates a feeling of paralysis, like a river which is frozen over or dammed up. On the other hand, large waves of water can overwhelm us, break boundaries and lay to waste the countryside. Many adults describe childhood moments where fear associated with water overwhelmed and consumed them.

THE BACKGROUND TO WATER IN CHINESE MEDICINE

Introduction

The Water Element consists of the concept of Water and its key associations. These are:

Organs   Kidney and Bladder
Spirit   Zhi — the mental-spiritual aspect of the Water Element
Colour   Blue
Sound   Groaning
Emotion   Fear
Odour   Putrid

These associations will be discussed in detail throughout the section. Familiarity with them will help us to recognize Water types and understand the connections between the Organ functions and mental processes described later.

Like the other organs described in this book the Kidneys and Bladder have mental and spiritual as well as physical functions. These two organs work closely together dealing with the storage of water in the body.

The Kidneys

The Kidney is called the Controller of Water and as such it oversees all of the fluids of the body. We are 83 per cent water so the Kidney's job is a significant one. Every system of our body involves fluids. As Controller, the Kidney influences whether we retain too much or too little fluid. When the warming Yang energy of the Kidney is weak, we retain fluids and can become cold and water-logged. When the cooling Yin energy of the Kidney is weak, we start to dry up, grow warmer and become wrinkled.

The Kidney also stores our 'Essence' which is our inherited energy. This Essence is the basis of our constitutional strength. It controls the longer-term cycles of growth and development, notably puberty, menopause and old age. When the Essence is strong, the bones of our skull will close properly, we will walk and talk on time, develop sexually and become fertile. We will sail through the menopause and grow old gracefully. When the Essence is weak, our life transitions may be less easy. Puberty and menstruation may be late, conception may be difficult and old age may arrive prematurely.

As well as controlling our growth and development, Kidney Essence also affects our brains. Kidney Essence is said to 'fill' our brains and help us to feel mentally intelligent and alert. Strengthening Kidney energy will often increase our alertness and ability to function from the mind as opposed to the feelings. This point will be significant later in the Water exercises. A famous ancient Chinese book which is called 'The simple questions' and which is over 2,000 years old says:[2]

> The Kidneys are responsible for the creation of power. Skill and ability stem from them.

The Kidneys and Water also house the 'Zhi' or the mental and spiritual aspect.

The Mental-Spiritual Aspect of Water

Zhi (pronounced 'jer') is translated as 'willpower', 'drive', 'ambition', or even 'the tendency towards something'. When we are healthy the Zhi allows us to experience a natural and unconscious ability to focus our minds and energy towards achieving our chosen ends. When the Kidneys are weak the person either develops more conscious determination or lapses into inertia.

Gerry, a Water type, describes:

> If I'm on a wave of action and I want to get there I'll do it even if I have to go under it or over it. Any problem that comes up I know if I keep on at it I'll slowly erode it. If I couldn't, it would be totally devastating.

Water types often appear to be determined people. The Water Element naturally gives us the ability to flow or move forward through the different stages of our lives. If this Element becomes imbalanced then Water types might not trust that this flow will happen naturally. They will therefore take control to make it happen. What previously would have been an unconscious drive to move forward becomes a conscious effort. This manifests in what we experience as the Water type's strong will and determination.

There is a limit, of course, to what the mind can do. Mike, another Water type, describes a weakened Zhi:

When I was young I'd work through my tiredness and I assumed it was a good thing to be indomitable and indefatigable — but I don't think that now. I used to be driven but not any more. Now I'm listless and couldn't care less.

The Bladder

The main significance of the Bladder Organ is its associated energy channel which runs alongside the spine and down the back of the legs. Many problems with the spine are treated using Bladder acupuncture points and the spine and legs are often where fear, the emotion of Water, is experienced. We speak of people who are fearless as having 'backbone' and those who are fearful as 'spineless'. Madelaine, a Water type, noticed:

One thing that happens to me, if I'm getting fearful or hurt I get a sensation up the back of my leg along the Bladder pathway. I've had it for 15 years now but I hadn't realized until two years ago that it followed that pathway. I get it when I'm anxious and upset.

The control of our urine is also associated with fear. Mike commented:

One way I know I'm scared is that my bladder tells me I'm not feeling easy and I want to pee a lot — I've learned then to look to see what's disturbing me.

THESE SYMPTOMS MAY ARISE WHEN THE KIDNEYS AND BLADDER ARE WEAK OR OBSTRUCTED

Some of these symptoms are more physical and some more mental or of the spirit. Chinese medicine being 'energetic' did not make this an important distinction.

Sore back, back pain and spinal problems. Too strong or the lack of willpower and inappropriate fearlessness. Fearfulness. Poor energy or lethargy. Weak or cold knees, swollen legs, excessive pale urination. Extreme restlessness, dizziness, tinnitus. Dark scanty urine. Night sweats. Ache in the bones. Thirst or a dry mouth. Excessive sexual desire. Infertility, a lack of sexual energy. Weak bones. Poor development in children. Poor concentration and memory. Hearing problems. Prematurely greying hair, falling hair or losing teeth.

Observable Signs of a Water Type

The following are some key signs which indicate that a person is a Water type:

+ A blue colour on the face (either pale blue or dark, almost black-blue) either under and to the side of the eyes or the black-blue around the mouth and more generally over the face.
+ A body odour for which the English translation is 'putrid ', which is almost sharp inside the nose and resembles the odour of chloride of lime mixed with urine or a stagnant pond.
+ A groaning sound in the voice where the natural variation up and down seems compressed resulting in a flat sound (imagine something frightening in the room with you and speaking very carefully so as not to disturb it).
+ A fearful or apparently fearless emotional state which will be referred to in a later section.

Posture, Gestures and Facial Expression

When we are afraid we may either shake or become very still. Water types in their everyday behaviours are often noticeably still. Also, when afraid, we may pull ourselves slightly back and sometimes Water types will carry this movement in their everyday posture.

Because the kidneys lie in the middle of the back, the spine of Water types may be slightly weaker than other areas of the body. If we observe the posture of a Water type we might sometimes see that they are slightly collapsed in the area of the lower back. This can cause a weak back or back pains. Here Dali tells us about her back:

My lower back is probably the major thing wrong with me. It has gone on the longest and shown the least sign of improvement. I get a dull ache when I'm tired towards the end of the day or when I've been standing a lot. It's worse when I exercise and I feel weak and cold there.

If a person is chronically afraid, the expression of fear can be imprinted on the face. Aside from the stillness mentioned above, which can be in the facial expression as well as the whole body, the eyes are the most likely part of the expression to reveal chronic fear. In the moment of fear, eyes can open wider and move from side to side and something of this response can be retained in non-threatening circumstances.

THE EMOTIONAL CAPACITY OF THE WATER ELEMENT

The Water Element produces certain capacities and we can describe them in the following way:

♦ Assessing risks
♦ Protecting ourselves appropriately

Assessing Risks

We might assess the security of our homes and buy burglar alarms, check the locks on our doors and windows and make sure we are properly insured. We might also join a local 'neighbourhood watch' scheme and find out what the local police are doing to protect the public.

When we have carried out these precautions, we might feel reassured, but perhaps not. If not, the perception of fear will still be there and we will continue to consider what could be done to ensure our safety.

The normal process we go through when assessing risks is that first we perceive a threat. This is usually accompanied by a feeling of fear. Secondly, we will carry out some activity to assess the potential risk then thirdly, take steps to ensure our ultimate safety. Finally, we will re-evaluate the situation.

This process of evaluation sometimes occurs within seconds and at other times takes much, much longer. We can only carry out this process with the support of a strong Water Element. It is a very skilful activity and explains the connection made in Chinese medicine between 'skill and cleverness' and the Kidneys.

Protecting Ourselves Appropriately

The Water emotion of fear alerts us to danger and is a necessary part of protecting ourselves. Indeed, survival requires a feeling of threat and an ability to respond. Thousands of years ago the threats were things such as dangerous animals, the attack of a rival tribe and harsh climatic conditions. Now, they are burglars, muggers, cars on the roads, rises in interest rates, or potential unemployment — dangers change over time.

If a threatening situation arises, such as an increase in muggings or burglaries in our area, most of us will look at the situation and examine how it might affect us. How can we avoid the potential violation?

EMOTIONS WE EXPERIENCE WHEN THE ABILITY IS IMPAIRED

The Water Element gives us the ability to assess risks and act appropriately. When this ability is diminished, we will have more ongoing experiences of:

♦ Anxiety and panic
♦ Paralysis
♦ Fear, apprehension and dread
♦ Phobias

We will talk about each of these in turn.

Anxiety and Panic

It is normal to feel afraid when we are under threat. If we feel threatened we do what we can to make ourselves feel safe. Water types may find it difficult to feel reassured. They may describe their fear in a variety of ways. Terror, apprehension, suspicion, dread, anxiety, trepidation or panic are some of the words used. Here Mike describes how he reacts when he becomes anxious:

> I'm scared most of the time to some degree or another. At times I may feel a contraction in my lower belly — I think it's to do with not knowing why I'm scared. If I know why I'm scared I'll have other symptoms. I'll feel an adrenalin rush — my heartbeat increases, my mouth goes dry and I need to pee.

When we are frightened we may become so scared that we wish to flee the situation as fast as possible. As we can't usually flee completely, in reality we might feel panicky, but not actually run off. Here Denise tells us how she reacts in certain situations:

> If I'm in a closed area and someone is walking towards me I immediately think, 'Will I be all right?' or I think, 'That person might be up to no good.' They're probably perfectly OK but I feel like running away.

REASSURANCE AND RECOVERY

Patients who are going to have an operation can feel fraught with anxiety and fear. It has been found helpful to give patients reassurance beforehand. Those patients who have their questions answered and are given clear guidelines about what to expect during their recovery period have been found to recover two to three days sooner than those who don't.[4]

Paralysis

Sometimes when Water types are frightened, they feel paralysed. Fear stops them from moving forward mentally or physically. New things seem too much of a risk. They may also find it takes them longer to achieve things than other people. Freda, a Water type, remembers being fearful and nervous from a very young age:

> I remember at five when I was learning to ride a bike. My father saw that I was nervous and wouldn't get on the bike and said, 'You'll never learn.' Any physical activity and I got very nervous. Swimming lessons were another example. I went to swimming lessons at nine years old and the same thing happened. My swimming teacher said, "She's so nervous she'll never learn." I was kind of paralysed.

A kind of paralysis can also develop from fear which is never processed. The fear gets stuck in the body, the mind is ever on the alert although not necessarily knowing for what, and the stillness described above is what we notice from the outside.

Fear, Apprehension and Dread

This is often a development from anxiety but it is usually more incapacitating. The threat we feel is often imagined and arising from our internally-generated perceptions — other non-Water types may be feeling cool and calm about the same situation. Dali describes her fears:

> My fears are ones that are off the scale rather than small worries and they're irrational too — too awful to even think about — a kind of dread. I was really

consumed with dread before going away to China, about going away, even though I wanted to go. My boyfriend couldn't understand me and then he started dreading it too so it was awful and it went on and on. Having been and come back I am not sure what it was about.

Under the surface many Water types feel scared much of the time. Sometimes they are conscious of it and sometimes not. Often they hide their fear beneath more 'acceptable' emotions, especially joy and laughter. Anger also often covers fear. Some Water types are not conscious of feeling frightened, but the fear is still stuck in their bodies. In this case they may have unexplained symptoms of the sort described on page 183. Uncovering their true feelings can be a major step to recovery. Looking at the 'Responses to the Big Issues' later in the chapter will help a Water type to clarify their real feelings.

FEAR AND OUR HEALTH

A study at Stanford University School of Medicine found that of women who had had heart attacks the ones who went on to have a second one were often those who were the most fearful. In many cases these women had chronic fears and might even have stopped driving, left their job or stopped going out.[5]

Phobias

Phobias are another type of fear which some people experience. A phobia is an intense and illogical fear which occurs in clearly defined situations, as if it is a one-off, learned response to specific stimuli. Phobias can arise in a huge variety of circumstances and common ones are fear of snakes, confined spaces, spiders or high places.

Not all people with phobias are Water types although some are. A person who has no major fears when they are not in their 'phobic' situation may not be a Water type. A person who has a phobia as well as a fearful disposition may be. The phobia can in this case be an indication of the Water type's inability to reassure her- or himself. A 'phobia cure' which has been successfully used for many people, is included in the next chapter.

Recognizing the Emotion of a Water Type in Everyday Life

Water types in everyday life tend to fall into two sorts: those who get frightened a lot and those that hardly ever seem to be frightened. The people who are frightened a lot are usually, if you know them well, not so hard to spot. An additional observation you can make is how they respond to reassurance.

For example, two friends of ours in the middle of winter were expressing concern, even fear, that they might succumb to a specific infectious illness. The illness was around, but catching it was by no means certain. As *objectively* as we could, we told them both what we knew about the likelihood of catching the disease, what could be done to avoid catching it and some other reasons why they might not catch it. One of them is not a Water type and she could *hear* the facts and reassurance we were relating. The other person is a Water type and she fidgeted, looked away, and interrupted several times with, 'Well, what about this', and 'what about that'. She was clearly *less able to hear*, which suggested that her fear was more deep-seated.

Curiously, the ears and hearing are associated with the Kidneys. Early deafness and recurring ear infections are often treated by strengthening the Kidneys. In the above example, the ability to hear information which might ameliorate the fear, definitely does depend upon the strength of the Kidneys.

The Water types who hardly ever seem to be frightened are harder to notice. If something frightening comes up, you may find yourself thinking, 'Well I would be frightened about this', and yet they seem casual if not cool. These are more likely to be people who do a lot of internal calculating and tend to avoid the conscious feelings of fear. Their approach to fear is described in a later section. Occasionally these people do things which are known to be frightening like parachuting, swimming with sharks and bungee jumping. They describe these as exhilarating or exciting, but not frightening.

BIG ISSUES AND UNANSWERED QUESTIONS FOR THE WATER TYPE

For any type, when typical negative experiences recur, certain issues become more important than others. The big issues for the Water type are:

♦ Needing to be safe
♦ Knowing the future is secure

♦ Being reassured

To say that these are the big issues is to say that in any situation, particularly ones of stress, the Water type will automatically be concerned with certain things. These include what needs to be done to make them feel safe from threats, determining who or what is reassuring to them and what will give them security in the future.

Another way of expressing the internal experience of someone whose Water is constitutionally impaired is that they begin to carry certain unanswered questions such as:

♦ Why is the world so dangerous?
♦ Will I ever be safe?
♦ Who can I trust?
♦ Where will I be safe?

For the non-Water type there are answers to these questions. For the Water type these questions keep recurring and to varying degrees do not get answered. The difficulties in finding answers can lead a Water type to develop various life patterns or strategies.

HOW WOULD YOU KNOW THAT YOUR FRIEND IS A WATER TYPE?

He or she might:
♦ look slightly blue around the eyes or have a dark, blackish face
♦ have a flat, almost compressed voice, especially when you would expect the tone to fluctuate more
♦ seem frightened a lot or not at all
♦ let you know, maybe inadvertently, that they think a lot about what might and what might not go wrong
♦ have jerky movements
♦ not put themselves forward even though they are right for the job
♦ often withdraw from a commitment

RESPONSES TO THE BIG ISSUES

The ways of coping which we will discuss next are a response to the Big Issues and Unanswered Questions. Given that these issues are important and the questions keep recurring these are the kinds of lifestyles or behaviours which a Water type might adopt to deal with their issues.

Not every Water type will use all of these strategies and there may be other variations which we have not observed. It is also possible for other types to behave in similar ways. In this case the behaviours might be less pronounced or have a different set of questions behind them.

The responses are:

♦ Taking risks
♦ Anticipating risks
♦ Questioning
♦ Fearing the worst
♦ Reassuring others

We will look at each of these in turn.

Taking Risks

We all face a number of risks every day. Crossing the street, having a bath, driving a car — there are many everyday, potentially dangerous situations. It might seem odd, therefore, to say that Water types, whose natural emotion is fear, will seek out risks. If they are already grounded in fear, why would they purposely put themselves into dangerous situations?

Some Water types have dealt with their fear by suppressing it. Others may perceive that they have a lack of fear. It is almost as if they need a larger stimulus than normal in order to experience the rush of adrenalin which normally accompanies fear. The feelings created by the challenge are experienced very positively and usually not labelled as fear. At the same time, purposefully putting themselves at risk 'proves' that they are brave and can cope with any situation.

These Water types are often called 'daredevils'. Some of their 'relaxations' might be rock climbing, parachuting, hang-gliding, wind surfing or deep sea diving. Some do these things in their spare time whilst others, like Evel Knievel, have made a profession out of it. A recent report in a newspaper showed photos of a professional daredevil riding a bicycle over a cliff and then parachuting down to rocks 450 feet below. He is quoted as saying:[6]

> Nothing comes close to that feeling when you are in mid-air and have made the choice and when on landing you realize that you have overcome your fear and succeeded in overcoming a huge mental challenge the situation has presented you with.

Interestingly, his stunt was funded by *Adrenalin* magazine!

Other Water types do 'daredevil' activities in their everyday lives. Here a colleague described a Water type she knows:

> She has the most scars of anyone I've ever met. She likes to go and walk along under the cliffs and get stuck in the tide and risk her neck. She really likes to live on the edge.

Even the most sensible of Water types may sometimes get into some risky situations as Freda and Dali explained. Freda told us:

> I'm usually very careful but I love speed. That's the buzz side. I'll drive too fast unless I'm being sensible. It makes me feel excited.

And Dali said:

> I suppose people say I'm adventurous. I would go off to India when I was younger or go hitch-hiking in Morocco on my own. As a woman, I felt fine, but others said I was foolish.

One of the secrets of some risk-takers is that they think they only do things that they know are ultimately safe. They like to be on the edge only as long as they are in control. Here Mike confirms this as he tells us:

> I used to be a bit reckless but it's never precipitated disasters. Even when I do something reckless I consider the worst possibility first. I never do anything blindly.

Sometimes things can go wrong for risk-takers, however. No amount of preparation was able to stop Richard Branson's balloon from capsizing when he tried to do his round the world trip.

Evel Knievel has broken 35 bones, been operated on 15 times and spent three years of his life in hospital. He was recently quoted as shrugging and saying, 'Hey, you have to pay the price for success.'[7]

Other Water types who appear to take chances are ones who love anticipating risks. Once again, we might wonder if they are really taking risks?

Anticipating Risks

Water types may respond by anticipating all possible hazards. They look carefully at what might happen in any given situation. This allows them to plan exactly how to behave and be prepared for all eventualities. Here Terry describes how he does this:

> I work out every possible thing that could go wrong so that if it does go wrong I am prepared for it. Somebody once said that I was the best person they knew to be with in a crisis. Because I just do what needs to be done. It's the anticipation that is the frightening thing, not the actual doing of it.

Gerry also likes to work out what to do:

> I usually work out every conceivable thing that could happen in a situation. To other people I seem intuitive but it just seems obvious to me because I anticipated what might happen.

Because of their need to anticipate what might happen in any situation many Water types can be very effective in achieving what they set out to do. We can couple the strong determination of the Water type with their ability to see ahead. The result is people who can set a goal then go forward and accomplish it. It doesn't matter how difficult the obstacles might be.

Many successful people who run businesses are Water types. Their ability to anticipate can lead them to outmanoeuvre all of their competitors. Richard Branson and Donald Trump, for example, are two well-known entrepreneurs who anticipate. Trump has described one property deal which was very profitable. Its essence was the anticipation of every potential difficulty and the off-loading of almost every potential loss.

Water types of this sort may appear to be more willing to take risks than some others types. We shouldn't be deceived. In reality they have thought through all the hazardous aspects of their ventures. The business deals they make are less of a gamble than they appear. They are so successful because the Water type won't follow through any really risky plans. Once they have minimized the danger the rest of the deal becomes an exciting adventure.

Questioning

Another way of assessing risks is by asking questions. Many Water types do this to try to make sure that people or situations are trustworthy. In reality when we are afraid it's hard to find any answers which are reassuring. As one Water type said to us, 'I don't think people really know the answers.' Sometimes the Water type's questions seem to be endless and the answers won't always satisfy them. Here Jean tells us why she asks questions:

> I'll ask questions to find out. That's the way I can get to trust that things will be all right. There's definitely a lot of thought about the future — the questions can impede me from moving forward if I never get an answer. Sometimes it drives everyone else mad. My friend says I'm like a terrier with a rag and in exasperation she finally says, 'Let it go Jean'.

Water types might finally be reassured but only after having probed through all possibilities. They may do this at least twice as fully as any of the other types would. Here Gerry tells us how she has done this by questioning two different people:

> I have a lack of trust and I'm continually having to question people to reassure myself. At the moment I've got a hernia and I'm booked in to see two people about it. I'm going to a hernia centre in London and the local specialist. I need to be reassured that the person locally is OK. I've learnt to make sure that inside myself I'm happy. *Double* reassurance makes me happy.

Another reason why Water types ask questions is to try to get beneath the surface of a person or a situation. For example, a person may be recommended to them as highly skilled in an area of work. They may be a trustworthy builder, a brilliant clinician or a good teacher. The recommendation will not be enough for a Water type who asks questions. They will ask many more probing questions to penetrate the superficial facade. In this way they will get to the truth about the person's real abilities.

When in the presence of a Water type of this sort, people might feel interrogated, or that they are under suspicion. To some degree this is true. If they pass the Water type's 'test', however, they will be respected and trusted by the Water type. That is until the next time — when they may be asked to prove once more that they are trustworthy. After all a lot can change in the space of a few weeks! Denise points out:

I find it very difficult to trust people lightly. They have to prove their trust to me or I have to ask lots of questions to make sure that I can then believe in them. If I don't feel I can trust them then I end up backing away. It's no good someone saying, 'He's a great man', 'He's been knighted', 'He's a doctor or consultant', or 'He's a headmaster'. There has to be a lot of questions and even more questions.

Once Water types have satisfied themselves about the integrity of the person they are 'assessing', they will feel more in control of their situation. This process of assessment which can take a few minutes for other types can be a much more lengthy process for a Water type. The understanding brought about through asking questions, however, gives them a greater feeling of safety and allows them to move on forward. One downside can be that the people being questioned or assessed may get the distinct feeling that they're being interrogated.

Some Water types don't overcome their fear or reassure themselves by asking questions. Some Water types fear the worst. In this case they may find their lives limited by their fear.

Fearing the Worst

When we are young we can easily become afraid and we then rely on our adult carers for reassurance. Children can feel scared in many situations. These can be things like a bad dream, a large dog or a school bully. A child's fears can easily be exaggerated out of all proportion to reality. Freda, for example, was afraid of many things as a child:

When I was young I was frightened of little things and I constantly thought, 'I wish I was braver'. Everyone else seemed not to be afraid but I was frightened of everything. I remember even having nightmares after seeing the film Bambi.

For most of us the reassurance our carers give us when we are young helps us to overcome or deal with scary situations. As long as we are not let down badly we will learn to reassure ourselves that our world is a safe place and that people can be trusted.

Many Water types, however, find it difficult to build this trust. They may be frightened when they think about the many things which could go wrong in the future. At the same time they may have no real reason to expect them to happen. If this is the case they may blow up their fear until it is out of all proportion to reality. Even the smallest of their anxieties can turn molehills into mountains. Madeleine, for example, has extreme fears about her health.

I blow things up if it's got to do with my health. I have a fear of what's going wrong with my body. I'm a health practitioner and sometimes I'm questioning my patients and they don't seem to be terribly frightened by things I'd be petrified of. The smallest things going wrong leads to the worst scenarios. In fact everyday I think, 'This is your last day'.

One of our Water-type patients had headaches. He was terrified that they were a brain tumour and didn't get them investigated. He began to plan dying and actually made a video of himself for his young daughter to play when he was gone. Once the headaches had stopped it was difficult for him to be sure they were gone.

Fear can lead us to imagine what others are thinking about us. We may limit ourselves because we are scared of what they think. Freda tells us how her fear caused her to give up something she enjoyed:

I recently started to learn bell ringing. I have a good touch and rhythm but I realized I'd take twenty times longer than anyone else. I could see people were getting impatient so I stopped. It was a combination of fearfulness and nervousness.

For others just seeing a potentially dangerous situation may cause them to exaggerate. In their mind it seems *extremely* dangerous even if they are really safe. Madeleine noticed:

When I'm up high my hands go clammy just thinking about it. I can't look over the edge and I imagine falling over. I once took the children up to the top of the Eiffel Tower and I just wanted to grab them and take them back down.

It is hard to live comfortably when we are in a continually fearful state. Sometimes we find it's easier to conceal what we're feeling beneath another emotion. This could be anger or laughter. At other times we may just pretend that we're not frightened at all.

Reassuring Others

In spite of the fear they feel on the inside some Water types can seem very reassuring on the outside. They have developed a stillness and an aura of safety and solidity. These steady rock Water types may work in jobs where their reassuring presence is held in high regard. They may be doctors, nurses or other health practitioners who have to reassure others even in a crisis. They could also work as security guards, lifeguards or in the police force where they need to be both brave and reassuring at the same time. In this case their suspicions and distrust can be put to good use in helping the general public. Other jobs which can also be appealing may be the armed forces such as the army, navy and air force.

Dali who is a health practitioner told us that others tell her she is reassuring:

> When I try to give reassurance and do it with words it doesn't work, but people say I have a reassuring presence. I have to acknowledge that people say I have it even though I might not feel it inside.

Earlier we mentioned that of all the emotions we experience, fear seems to be the one we hide the most. Many Water types may be terrified inside but be reassuring, calm and brave on the outside. Denise is an example of someone like this.

> People will say to me, 'you're brave', but I don't notice it. What may look brave to them can be terrifying to me. I couldn't go to the top of the Eiffel Tower and no way would I bungee jump. To me these are things that don't need to be done. If on the other hand something has to be faced I will just do it even though I'm frightened.

Most Water types find that they have a mixture of the strategies which we have described above. It may seem to be a contradiction that they can be both very calm and brave but fearful and nervous too. Here Gerry describes being both frightened and fearless:

I get fearful in physical ways like I have a fear of flying. It's really being out of control that is so difficult. I can climb and I drive very fast. I'm a terrible passenger but when I'm driving I'm very good. A few years ago I went to a place in France which is called the Pont du Gard. It's a huge and very high aqueduct. At the top it's nine feet wide and every so often there are nine-inch holes through the paving stones so there was a huge drop below. Others were frightened but I could walk over it with no fear as I was in control. I couldn't go bungee jumping as I'd be out of control.

Gerry says she remains unafraid as long as she is in control of the situation she finds herself in. Once out of control she may easily become terrified. This helps to explain the swing between the two sides of the emotion.

VIRTUES AND VICES OF A WATER TYPE

Depending on the health of the Water type, the strategies produce both virtues and vices. Some of the virtues are:
♦ A highly developed capacity to assess what is safe
♦ Strong determination in the face of difficulties
♦ Courage in a crisis
♦ The capacity to anticipate difficulties and proceed with safety.
Some of the vices are:
♦ Excessive fear
♦ False bravado in what seem like scary situations
♦ A failure to appreciate real and obvious danger.

A FAMOUS WATER TYPE — PRESIDENT JOHN F KENNEDY[8]

Few Americans have been as widely revered as the famous Water type President, John F Kennedy. It is said that courage and death were two of the enduring themes of his life. 'Courage' was said to be the virtue he most admired. His brother Robert said that this, 'could be physical courage such as a man under army fire, or men who suffered pain or who climbed mountains but also moral courage'.

Later Kennedy wrote that moral courage is the 'Courage of the man who does what he must — in spite of personal consequences, in spite of obstacles, danger and pressures.' Later still he wrote a book called *Profiles in Courage* which gave inspirational examples of courage within the senate.

His life was a mixture of many of the strategies of a Water type. He was both inclined to take risks and at the same time he had a finely-tuned ability to 'anticipate risks'. This was shown clearly by the way he dealt with the Cuban missile crisis. As president, he also had the ability to 'be reassuring'. His very presence seemed to reassure people that they were in safe hands. We can speculate, however, that anyone who so admired courage must have had his own personal struggle against fear.

He joined the navy in 1941 and was noted for his calm and bravery. He was said to have saved a man by gripping the end of his life jacket between his teeth, something he later described in true Water type style as an 'interesting experience'. He was awarded a medal for his heroism.

He campaigned tirelessly for a seat in the Senate and during campaigning in 1951 was taken seriously ill and had to walk with crutches. This was never made public. When he came to the door of the hall where he was due to give a speech he handed over the crutches, threw his shoulders back and marched down the aisle as if he was not in pain. He was carrying out an act of bravery of the sort he had always so admired.

In typical Water type fashion he was a hard worker and campaigner. In the last few days of his presidential campaign he survived on only four hours' sleep a night in spite of being in frail health.

In fact, it is now known that John Kennedy was a sickly child — this was covered up during his presidential campaigns. Chinese medicine understands that the spine is closely connected with the Kidney and Bladder Organs, so it is not surprising to hear that he was born with an unstable spine. His back progressively deteriorated throughout his life and caused him to have two operations. He also had to wear a special corset.

In 1947 he was diagnosed as having another serious illness which is closely associated with an imbalance in the Kidneys. This is called Addison's disease which causes impaired functioning of the adrenal glands. In order to survive he had to take cortico-steroid drugs. His now-so-famous sexual appetite can at least in part be attributed to these drugs.

Interestingly, his presidency was marked by a series of economic and security crises. We could speculate that some of these maybe could have been avoided if he had not been such a risk taker. The Cuban missile crisis was one of the most famous and he has been described as standing 'eye-ball to eye-ball' with the Russian president who had been building up missiles in Cuba. Fortunately, the Russian president stepped down, avoiding a third world war.

We can speculate about what would have happened had the president not been a Water type. Would another president have caved in to the Russians and not taken the risk or would he have prevented the situation from escalating into a crisis? We will never know. The Western world went into mourning when he was assassinated in 1963, three years after being elected president.

GOLDEN RULES FOR WATER TYPES

♦ It is natural to notice threats, feel fear, assess the risks and act accordingly.
♦ Anticipating and being careful is important *and* allow for enjoying yourself now.
♦ Notice whether what you think of as a risk is perceived by others differently, for example, as an opportunity.
♦ Find out when it is useful to pull back and anticipate and when it is useful to engage — discriminate between the two.
♦ When you are concerned about something in the future, imagine going beyond that point in time and look back.

Notes

1 Weiger, L, 1965: *Chinese Characters*; page 287
2 From the *Huang Qi Nei Jing* or *Yellow Emperor's Classic of Internal Medicine*. There are two parts to this book. This is in the part called the *Su Wen* or *Simple Questions*. There are many translations.
3 Larre, Claude, Schatz, Jean, Rochat de la Vallee, Elisabeth, 1986: *Survey of Traditional Chinese Medicine*; Institut Ricci, Paris, and Traditional Acupuncture Foundation, Columbia, Maryland, page 176.
4 Daniel Goleman: *Emotional Intelligence*; Bloomsbury Publishing, Chapter 11, page 174.
5 Daniel Goleman: *Emotional Intelligence*; Bloomsbury Publishing, Chapter 11, page 182.
6 *Daily Mail*, Saturday 23 May, 1998
7 *Sunday Times*, New Review Section, June, 1998
8 The information about President Kennedy is taken from Reeves, Thomas C (editor), 1990, and Reeves, Thomas C, 1991.

Chapter 11

EXERCISES FOR WATER TYPES

INTRODUCTION

The exercises in this chapter are aimed at enabling Water types to find a better emotional balance. Some useful goals for Water types are:

- To learn to *dissociate* from scary situations
- To learn to re-experience somatized feelings of fear
- To reassure themselves
- To overcome their excessive fear

USING THE EXERCISES

We suggest that you read an exercise through before you start it. All of the exercises are laid out in a similar style. Following the *introduction*, we tell you approximately *how long* it will take to complete. Obviously some of you will take more time and others less. The exercises are then divided into stages. They start with:

- the *purpose* of the exercise and then
- the *process* or the steps of the exercise.

The theme of each step is in bold so that you have a summary. At the end of some exercises we have a section called *'matters arising'*. Here we discuss issues which could come up while you do the exercise.

THE EXERCISES FOR WATER TYPES

♦ Dissociating from our fears
♦ Transforming our fear
♦ Reclaiming our lost sensations of fear
♦ Reassuring ourselves
♦ Dealing with one-off fears and phobias
♦ Qigong Dragon swimming exercise
♦ A Qigong exercise — the hula hoop

EXERCISE 1 — DISSOCIATING FROM OUR FEARS

Introduction

As a child Paul was anxious and frightened and he continued into adult life feeling more or less the same. He took ages to move in with Henrietta, anticipating endless possible disadvantages and repetitively discussing each of them with her. After four years of near-wedlock, Henrietta finally said 'now or never'. Paul was frightened she would truly find someone else and he finally committed himself.

He approached the following exercise with interest as he could not quite imagine what it would be like to extract himself from fear and consider a situation more rationally. It took him some time to do the exercise. By doing it Paul said that he had gained something he had never had before. This was a way of stepping out of his fear and finding a place within himself from which he could operate without the confusion and indecision that fear engendered.

Time needed: 15–20 minutes.

Purpose

Fear is often a useful indicator that something is threatening. If the fear has too strong a grip, it stops us from acting appropriately in the light of the threat. The purpose of this exercise is to differentiate two different internal perspectives and to learn to move from the former to the latter. Briefly, these two positions are:

♦ 'Dissociation' is a detached position from where we are looking at both ourselves and our situation as if we were an impartial observer.

♦ 'Association' or an attached position is when we are rooted in ourselves and are seeing things from our own point of view.

'Association' and 'dissociation' will be used in later exercises so what is learned here will also be useful later.

Process

1 **Find a situation where you are frightened or anxious about what might happen.** Examples of this could be:
   ♦ Fear of doing something new
   ♦ Anxiety about sitting an exam or giving a talk
   ♦ Fear of what others might say about you
   ♦ Being frightened about what might happen to someone close
2 **Find a place where you know you have time and will not be disturbed. Mark out two positions on the floor.** One is your own, associated, position, the second is the position where you can be dissociated from both yourself and the rest of the situation.
3 **Briefly step into the associated position.** This is where you are experiencing the feelings of fear. The stepping in is to check that these feelings are real.

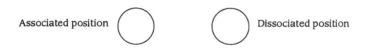

Associated position   Dissociated position

Figure 14: ASSOCIATED AND DISSOCIATED POSITIONS

4 **Now step into the dissociated position.** In this position you can look at yourself and the imagined situation from an outside perspective, as if you were someone else.
5 **From this position, notice certain aspects about yourself feeling fearful.** Now notice how *you* look in the image? If your name is Paul, you can say:
   ♦ What is Paul's posture like?
   ♦ Is Paul tense or relaxed?
   ♦ Is he well grounded on the Earth or slightly above it?
   Next, check how he is feeling by asking:

♦ How is the Paul I am looking at feeling?

Make sure that Paul is the one who is frightened and that you are not. If the dissociated 'you' is feeling the same fear as Paul, then transfer the feeling to the 'you' in your image. You might say, 'I allow these feelings to go back to Paul', that is the Paul that you are seeing. Continue, only when the fear feelings are fully and completely in the associated position of Paul, not in you. If the feelings have remained in you to even a small degree, then you might move your image of 'Paul' a little further away and say 'The Paul over there is the one who is afraid.'

In the dissociated position, if you are not feeling frightened, what should you be feeling? Some possibilities are: curious, compassionate or benevolent.

6 **Say out loud to the Paul in the image:** 'Paul, whatever feelings you are having are OK. They are just a starting point and they may be useful and they may not be useful. It is fine right now to have those feelings.'

Notice any changes to your image as you say this.

7 **As you did in step 3, walk over and** *briefly step into the associated position.* Notice how you are feeling and while you are there, say to yourself: 'I am feeling ... and it is fine for me to have these feelings right now and they may be useful or they may not be.'

Then step out of the associated position. Briefly compare your feelings there with how they were in step 3.

8 **Step back into the dissociated position and repeat step 6, but noticing any differences from the first time.** Note down any differences to your fear.

EXERCISE 2 — TRANSFORMING OUR FEAR

Introduction

Paul carried on with this exercise. He had believed, as most of us do, that feelings just occur or take us over — that we do not have much say in how we feel. What he discovered in this exercise was some of the ways he made himself frightened. When one particular fear almost completely disappeared as the result of what he did, he laughed out loud with delight and surprise.

Time needed: 15–20 minutes.

Purpose

The purpose of this exercise is to discover how we create and increase some of our fears by what we do in our head — which in turn can give us some control over the fear.

Process

1 **Find a situation which makes you frightened or anxious**. This might be the same situation you used in Exercise 1.
2 **Go back to the dissociated position.** See the situation as you imagine it will be *just before it happens*. If you have had a break you may need to do steps 1–5 of the previous exercise again.
3 **Now step into the associated position. Remain at the time just before the fear has happened. Say to yourself 'What do I do on the inside to create this fear?'** Before the fear appears you will be creating images, feelings or hearing sounds which bring on the feelings. Notice what you do, just before the fear appears. For example, people may discover just before the fear starts that they hear a parent's warning voice or see a quick flash of an image in which the people are huge, have enormous eyes and are staring at them critically — not unlike the scenes that might appear in horror movies. We stay afraid by keeping these voices or pictures just outside our consciousness.
4 **Now go back to the dissociated position and try changing the voice or the picture in a variety of ways.** Some suggestions are:
   ◆ Change the location of the voice so that it comes from another direction or so that you hear it in the other ear.
   ◆ Change the tone of the voice so it is chipmunkish or Donald Duckish.
   ◆ Change the location of the picture from one side to the other, from higher to lower or vice versa, or from nearer to further away.
   ◆ Make the picture fuzzier or clearer, darker or lighter.
   ◆ Change the picture to either colour or black and white.
   ◆ Make yourself or any other people in the picture more normal, for example, make others and yourself the same size, put yourself on the ground if you are floating.
6 **Once you have made the changes, step into the associated position again and experience the event which made you afraid.** If the fear has gone or really reduced, you have learned something about how you can create

fearful images and make yourself frightened. If you have done this once, then it is likely you do it as a pattern. Learn from this and be prepared to wonder what you do to create other instances that are frightening.

Matters Arising

It may be helpful for someone else to ask the questions in this exercise and it may take a few attempts to discover what you are doing before you feel afraid.[1]

EXERCISE 3 — RECLAIMING OUR LOST SENSATIONS OF FEAR

Introduction

Jeffrey is a Water type who could not remember the last time he was afraid. In his work he is good at anticipating and assessing risks and in his personal life he has the best mortgage, the cheapest car insurance, the best pension plan and very good home and contents insurance.

He has a few physical symptoms and he has been curious about the relationship between his fear and these symptoms. After doing the following exercise the recommended number of times, he said he had begun to understand what fear is and how he has reacted to it. At the same time his symptoms have eased.

Time needed: 10–15 minutes.

Purpose

This exercise is to help us to find and resolve our fearful feelings. It is designed for Water types who have developed an automatic and dissociated response to fear. This tends to cut out their conscious and associated awareness of the feeling of fear. These Water types rarely say they feel fear and can sometimes even seem rather fearless or even reckless. The contact with and the release of the fear can affect physical symptoms. Tension caused by unresolved fear can weaken the Kidneys and strain our adrenal glands — the organs of fright or flight. Unless resolved, this tension can store up ill health for the future.

Process

1 **Find a quiet comfortable place to do this exercise.** **Locate some feelings of discomfort which you think might be associated with fear,** but you don't understand why they are there. This can be any sensation and could include a tight feeling in your abdomen, a tension in your stomach or chest area, a recurring fearful thought, sweaty palms or a back ache.

2 **Now tune in to the sensation or body area and feel it for a while.** Give yourself time to let the sensations become clearer inside yourself. Take all the time you need. If your mind wanders, just bring it back to the sensations of body area.

3 **Say 'Hello' to the feeling.** When you have done this notice how your body responds. The feeling may change slightly or you may relax or settle a bit inside. This is because you have started to give the feeling some recognition.

4 **Now find a word, sentence or image to describe the sensation.** It may take some time to find the right word. Try out different words or images until you find one which is an exact 'fit'. When you find a word that fits the sensation, you will often feel the sensation change slightly.

Examples of words or sentences could be:

♦ Dread
♦ Jittery and anxious
♦ Feeling heavy and uneasy
♦ Lifeless and frozen

Whatever words arise do not judge them. Just let them be.

5 **Now shuttle between feeling the sensation and saying the word or sentence** which you have found. Keep moving backwards and forwards between the two. While you do this you might experience more changes to the sensation. Sometimes the word will change and a new and better one will appear. Continue shuttling between the sensation and the new word, phrase or image for a few minutes before going on to the next stage.

6 **Ask questions and find answers.** Ask yourself this question: 'What is the reason for this feeling which I call ...'

For example, if you are feeling tension in your stomach and the word which arises is 'Dread' then ask yourself, 'What is the reason for this feeling which I call dread?' Now wait until an answer arises. A response which arises immediately is not usually the true answer. Wait until an answer arises from deep within yourself. Write down the answer.

7 **Thank the sensation for any new understanding and knowledge.** If you wish to return, let it know that you will come back later. Consider what you have learnt about the sensation. You may be surprised by the response you received but it may also have provided you with new insights.

Matters Arising

Only with ten or more interactions with various sensations, will you be able to evaluate the benefits.

EXERCISE 4 — REASSURING OURSELVES

Introduction

Henrietta said that she had spent years immersed in feelings of anxiety and fright and wanted to know what people who didn't do this actually did. 'How do people deal with all the threats that arise one after another?' This exercise gave her the basis for a new mental habit. It took her some time to install the habit, but she says now, 'I may be a novice, but when something frightening arises — and they still do — at least I know what to do!'

Time Required: Once through this exercise will require roughly 20 minutes. It will take more time to make it a habit.

Purpose

This exercise is to teach Water types to reassure themselves when they are afraid.

Because Water types often have deep fears, the ability to reassure themselves may take some practice. It is worth persevering, however, as this habit or skill can be useful for a lifetime.

Process

1 **Think of something you are anxious about,** frightened about, maybe even despairing about. For instance it could be a health problem, it could be to do with your state of mind, or to do with financial security, or the welfare of your children.

2 **Now, as you learned in Exercise 1, dissociate from the problem and**

see yourself having the concern or anxiety or fear. Remember step 5 specifically. Use this state throughout the exercise.

3 **Use a piece of paper and divide it down the centre into two columns.** Put at the top of the left hand column 'Satisfactory Resolution', and at the top of the right hand column 'Unsatisfactory Resolution'. On the first line, put in the left hand column what would count as a satisfactory resolution. Be specific and make sure what you write satisfies the following criteria:

♦ You have stated the resolution positively, something you can include in your life, not something you want to exclude. This step may require some thought and may take a few minutes.

♦ You will have simple evidence for knowing when you have achieved the satisfactory resolution.

♦ The resolution is, if necessary, broken down into stages or smaller stages.

In the right hand column, write what is an unsatisfactory resolution.

MY PROBLEM	
Satisfactory solution	Unsatisfactory solution
Positive How will happen Specific	
Evidence why this might happen	Evidence why this might happen

Figure 15: REASSURING OURSELVES

4 **Now write down all the factors which are currently evidence for you that the particular resolution, satisfactory or unsatisfactory, is likely to arise.** Write this below the satisfactory and the unsatisfactory headings.

When considering what is likely to happen, you can use any information you wish. However, there is one sort of information which you are forbidden to use in this exercise. This is how you are feeling. You can assume, whether it is true or not, that your feelings are distorting your view. When we feel 'up' we often feel good about the future. When we feel 'down' we may then feel bad about the future. In this exercise how you feel doesn't count. Use your head, *as if the only thing you cared about was to be objective.* If you can, find several bits of evidence to put on each side of your paper.

5   **Now, imagine that someone you do not know has come to you with this piece of paper.** Assume his name is Alan. Pretend Alan has just handed it to you and asks for your opinion about what to do. Now go to a dissociated position on Alan's behalf (see exercise 1). Imagine that you are Alan and as Alan you are looking at yourself and anyone else who is in involved in the issue.

Ask yourself some useful questions:

♦ What is the worst case scenario in this situation?

♦ What can Alan do to improve the chances of a satisfactory resolution?

♦ Has Alan faced something like this before and if so how did he get through it?

♦ What other resources should Alan use?

♦ Who else's experience can Alan draw on?

♦ What is the best way for Alan to proceed?

♦ What emotional support can Alan get?

6   **Based on the answers you received, write down three things you can do and act on them promptly.** If necessary, repeat the exercise with the same situation again.

Do this exercise at least once a day for two to three weeks. This may sound a lot, but if this exercise is relevant for you, you need to practise, practise and practise some more. As you do this exercise, notice the gradual improvement you feel inside.

EXERCISE 5 — DEALING WITH ONE-OFF FEARS AND PHOBIAS

Introduction

Marion had a phobia about birds. She could not, for example, walk into squares in London because of the pigeons. She said that she would tighten up in the shoulders and chest, find her heart racing and feel panicky. Even talking about encountering birds started to bring on these feelings. She thought the phobia came from a time when she was very young, but her memory was not clear. She was not generally a frightened person so she got someone to take her through the following exercise. At the time she thought she felt a bit different, but two days later she had a chance to encounter a group of pigeons. She was puzzled by the absence of her response and then delighted.

Time required: 15 minutes.

Purpose

This exercise is one of the most effective we know for dealing with one-off fears and phobias. It will benefit anyone who has a phobia. We have put it in with the exercises for Water types as it will also enable Water types to deal with specific fears which interfere with their lives.

Examples of some of the phobias which people may experience are fears of confined spaces, going over bridges, heights, birds or specific insects such as spiders. Phobias such as these are often caused by a one-off event. For instance, a person who was trapped in a lift at the age of five subsequently suffered from claustrophobia or the fear of confined spaces. In other ways he was not an exceptionally fearful person. (For more on phobias see Chapter 10, page 188.)

Process

1 **Specify what it is that you are afraid of.** Either use an example of it, for instance, getting into a confined space, or, preferably, use a memory of the original event, for example, being trapped in a lift.

2 **Turn your mind to something else so that you are starting in a neutral state.**

3 **Imagine that you are in a cinema.** You are sitting in the back row, looking at the screen waiting for a film which is about to begin. The film will be about you.

4 **Move up to the projection booth** from where you can see yourself both in the cinema watching the screen and also on the screen itself. Check that you are feeling comfortable. If you are not, stop and do something else until you feel comfortable again.

5 **From the projection booth, watch yourself watching a black and white film of either the event that caused the fear or an example of it happening now.** You are in this film. Run the film so that it begins before the incident which caused distress. Carry on running the film until the end of the incident. At this point you should feel safe and comfortable again. When the film stops it will still have a black and white picture.

If you begin to feel uncomfortable while this film of you is showing, stop, get comfortable and start again. Make sure that you are in the projection booth, watching yourself watching the film. You will only become uncomfortable if you start to feel the feelings that the you in the film is experiencing. Remember that these are not your feelings but belong to the 'you' in the film.

6 **Now, step into the black and white still picture at the end of the film (where you are safe). Turn everything into full colour and quickly run the film backwards.** This is as if your time machine had gone into reverse. Although you know the film is being played in reverse the speed at which it is playing prevents you from identifying any part of the film. End up in the safe position where it all started. You can now step out of the film and watch it being played fast forward at high speed. Jump in once again and play it fast backwards. Repeat this three times. You should end in a comfortable place at the end of the film.

7 **Test what you have done.** Imagine some situations in which you would previously have felt distressed. As soon as possible go to the situation itself and discover what happens! The chances are that you will no longer find it disturbing.

QIGONG DRAGON SWIMMING EXERCISE[3]

Introduction

Louisa is a Water type who felt tired a lot, hated the cold and was overweight. Her Kidneys were weak and she practised the following exercise two to three minutes a day at first, but gradually worked up to two sessions of five minutes each. Over three months she lost weight around her waist and from her legs and felt much less tired and better able to deal with the cold.

Time needed: 5 minutes per day building to 10 minutes.

Purpose

The movement of this exercise strengthens the Kidneys, the spine and the lower abdomen.

Process

1 **Stand with your feet together.** From your hips, bounce gently up and down. Feel how your weight travels down from your hips to your feet which are solid on the floor. Tuck in your pelvis so that your back is straight.

2 **Hold the palms of the hands pushed tightly together with the fingertips pointing upwards.** Move from the lower abdomen. Move the hands in three circles going up and down the body to create a spiralling movement (see Figure 16).

3 **This exercise can be practised either gently or more vigorously.** To gain the most benefit from this exercise practise it regularly.

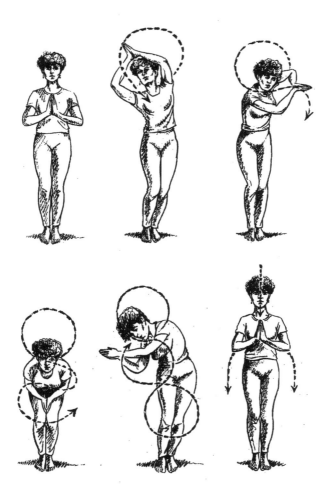

Figure 16: QIGONG DRAGON SWIMMING EXERCISE

QIGONG EXERCISE — THE HULA HOOP[4]

Introduction

Gregory is a Water type who described himself as 'depressed'. What this meant was that he spent time on his own, often thinking about being with others, but feeling too wary about actually making contact with them. He committed himself to doing this exercise for at least five minutes a day — along with working through the previous exercises. After two months he was spending at least three nights a week with friends and making more contact with his colleagues at work. He said for him this was 'a great change'.

Time needed: 5–10 minutes a day.

Purpose

This gentle exercise will strengthen your Kidneys.

Process

1 **Stand comfortably with your feet shoulders' width apart.**
2 **Rub your hands together until they feel warmer and place them on your back, over the kidneys** (see Figure 17). If necessary, consult an anatomy book to be clear about exactly where your kidneys are located. If you can't get the palm of your hands exactly on your kidneys, put them as close as you can. Imagine energy going from your palms into your kidneys. Repeat rubbing your hands together making them warmer and replace on your back.
3 **After a few minutes, keeping your hands on your back, begin to rotate your hips as if rolling a hula hoop around them,** 20 circles clockwise, then 20 counter-clockwise. As you circle your hips, imagine that fresh energy is cleansing and strengthening your kidneys. Keep the circle as smooth as you can.

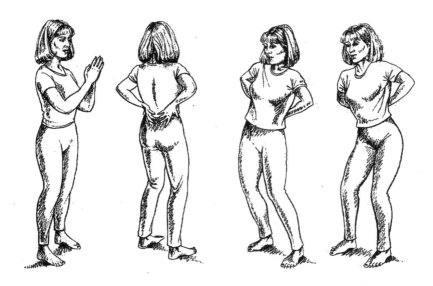

Figure 17: QIGONG EXERCISE — THE HULA HOOP

Matters Arising

As a rough guide, if exercising for five minutes, you could spend half the time rubbing your hands and holding them on your kidneys and the other half with your hands on your kidneys circling your hips. Get the movements correct first and then add in the impression that fresh energy is cleansing and strengthening your kidneys.

Notes

1   There is a good example of this approach being used in Andreas, Connirae and Andreas, Steve, 1989: *Heart of the Mind*; pages 1–3.
2   Andreas, Connirae and Andreas, Steve, 1989: *Heart of the Mind*; pages 55–71.
3   Zhizhong, Bian, 1987: *Daoist Health Preservation Exercises;* China Reconstructs Press, page 54.
4   See Kit, Wong Kiew, 1997: *Chi Kung For Health and Vitality*; pages 41–3.

Chapter 12

THE FIVE TYPES – WHICH TYPE AM I?

INTRODUCTION

The purpose of this chapter is to help you to clarify which type you are.

At the moment, you may be in varying stages of uncertainty. Some of you may have read through the chapters describing the types and thought you were each one that you studied! In this case you may now have no idea which type you are. On the other hand, you may have recognized your type immediately or narrowed it down to one or two. Recognizing yourself by reading through the type and saying, 'Yes, this is me!' is probably the best way of discovering your type. However, you may have turned directly to this chapter in order to fill in the questionnaire.

A few of you will not like questionnaires and no questionnaire is a perfect instrument. This questionnaire was constructed using people who know their types. These people answered a very long questionnaire and their answers were correlated with their type. Thus we were able to choose a smaller number of questions which we believe distinctively indicate the different types.

Because we are a combination of the Five Elements, you will gain points for all the different types. A slightly higher score is a sufficient indication of your type. If two types are higher than the other three, then consider that the highest scoring one is very probably your type, but that the second one might be. At worst, the questionnaire, will only narrow down the search. After completing the questionnaire, read through both the relevant chapter on the type(s) and the exercises. Then you can ponder what we have called the Big Issues, Unanswered Questions and the Responses to the Big Issues before making your final decision.

There are two things worth remembering. Because people have varying degrees of awareness of who they are, it is natural to have some doubts whether a particular type is really you. In addition, because there are only five types and therefore a lot of variety in the way a type can manifest, it is also natural that not everything we have put down about a type applies to you.

USING THE QUESTIONNAIRE

The questionnaire is straightforward. You will read seventy-five statements about symptoms, attitudes or values. You are asked to:

- ◆ 'strongly agree', in which case put a '3' in the adjacent box
- ◆ 'just agree', in which case you put a '2' in the adjacent box
- ◆ 'agree only a small amount', in which case you put a '1' in the adjacent box.
- ◆ 'do not agree at all', in which case you put a '0' in the adjacent box.

You might interpret the words which express your degree of agreement somewhat differently from someone else. This doesn't matter as long as you are consistent throughout the whole questionnaire. Because it is sometimes hard to keep the scoring table in mind, on each page there is a reminder of how many points to record according to your level of agreement.

When you have completed the questionnaire, transfer your answers to the grid at the end and total up the scores for each type. It is preferable not to look at the grid before answering the questions.

IF ALL ELSE FAILS

If you end up with no idea what your constitutional type is, you could consult an acupuncturist who uses this diagnosis in her or his practice. To find out how to do this, consult the Appendix.

QUESTIONNAIRE

HOW TO SCORE	
Strongly agree	3
Just agree	2
Agree only a small amount	1
Do not agree at all	0

☐ 1. I can get dizzy or lightheaded when standing up.

☐ 2. I am often anxious and restless.

☐ 3. I often have loose bowels.

☐ 4. I am easily disappointed or offended, but rarely show it.

☐ 5. People may think I am intuitive, but I actually do a lot of thinking ahead and working things out.

☐ 6. When someone is obviously being treated unfairly, I am often willing to stand up for the under-dog or the oppressed.

☐ 7. I laugh or giggle a lot.

☐ 8. At times, I have difficulty taking information in.

☐ 9. As soon as things do not work out, I think it is better to cut your losses and move on.

☐ 10. In a crisis, compared to others I am cool and can take charge.

☐ 11. Correctness and fairness are important, but difficult to achieve in practice.

☐ 12. I can be hurt by one simple comment and nevertheless hide my feelings.

☐ 13. I enjoy helping others and being useful to them.

☐ 14. I hate losing even small things.

☐ 15. I have weak or sore knees.

☐ 16. I often get really wound up and frustrated over issues.

☐ 17. Being happy is not the only thing in life, but it is close to the top of my list.

☐ 18. I feel worse with damp or humid weather.

☐ 19. I think, and others confirm this, that I am not emotionally expressive.

☐ 20. I sometimes get puffiness and dark bags under my eyes.

☐ 21. I prefer not to be supervised or overseen by others.

☐ 22. I look forward to socializing with or working with people.

☐ 23. I often feel tired and heavy.

☐ 24. I think a lot of my good qualities are not appreciated or recognized.

☐ 25. Having sex makes me tired/weak afterwards.

☐ 26. I often feel like rebelling or challenging authority or conventional wisdom.

☐ 27. I think I am over excitable.

☐ 28. I will often worry about things, even when I cannot do anything practical about them

☐ 29. I easily catch colds.

☐ 30. All I have to do is think about certain situations to make me feel concerned or even frightened.

☐ 31. I get blurred vision or tired eyes.

☐ 32. If my close relationships are not stable, I am not stable.

HOW TO SCORE	
Strongly agree	3
Just agree	2
Agree only a small amount	1
Do not agree at all	0

☐ 33. I am frequently worried and concerned about something.

☐ 34. My voice is a bit weak.

☐ 35. No one can reassure me – I need to reassure myself.

☐ 36. I enjoy organizing and structuring any situation.

☐ 37. I can easily doubt that someone loves me or cares for me.

☐ 38. I have some problems in balancing others and my own needs.

☐ 39. I appreciate it if I can do more and better than others.

☐ 40. I often need to assess a situation and check out whether I am safe.

☐ 41. On issues to do with who is responsible for what, I either have very specific views or I am completely easy.

☐ 42. A hurtful look or comment can leave me feeling very sad.

☐ 43. I sometimes do not digest well.

☐ 44. I frequently cough, with or without phlegm.

☐ 45. I am easily frightened, have phobias or get paranoid.

☐ 46. I have difficulty digesting fatty foods or a poor tolerance of alcohol.

☐ 47. I can go up and down a lot, loving things at one moment and feeling miserable the next.

☐ 48. I have an eating disorder or some irregularity of appetite.

☐ 49. I tend to set high standards for myself – and others.

☐ 50. I think people often tell you 'everything will be fine' and it won't.

☐ 51. It is better for me to be in control and have the power in any situation rather than be cooperating with and depending upon others.

☐ 52. I love safe, heart-felt contact with others.

☐ 53. My abdomen bloats after eating.

☐ 54. I always notice when people start talking about getting the best quality this and the best quality that.

☐ 55. I am good at looking ahead and anticipating what might go wrong.

☐ 56. I can get frustrated and wound up.

☐ 57. I often get tongue-tied or mix up my words.

☐ 58. I can be hungry, even after eating.

☐ 59. Finding your spiritual path is twenty times as important as just having a good time.

☐ 60. I tend to believe the world is a dangerous place and one needs to be careful.

HOW TO SCORE	
Strongly agree	3
Just agree	2
Agree only a small amount	1
Do not agree at all	0

☐ 61. I get muscle tightness or tension.

☐ 62. One of the best things in life is contact with other people.

☐ 63. I sometimes feel muzzy headed or can't think well.

☐ 64. Whatever I do, I prefer to do it as well as and preferably a lot better than others.

☐ 65. It takes me a while to really trust someone.

☐ 66. It makes me angry to see others being treated unjustly or unfairly.

☐ 67. Closeness with people is important to me.

☐ 68. I will sometimes worry about getting my needs met.

☐ 69. I easily get short of breath.

☐ 70. I urinate frequently and sometimes with some urgency.

☐ 71. My nails are weak or split.

☐ 72. I could be anxious and insecure about going to a party which I wanted to go to, but where there would be a lot of people I don't know – and I might not go.

☐ 73. Food and cooking are very important to me.

☐ 74. My breathing is shallow and sometimes weak.

☐ 75. People need to prove to me that they are trustworthy – I don't just believe it.

Q No.	Score	Q No.	Score	Q No.	Score	Q. No.	Score	Q.No.	Score
1		2		3		4		5	
6		7		8		9		10	
11		12		13		14		15	
16		17		18		19		20	
21		22		23		24		25	
26		27		28		29		30	
31		32		33		34		35	
36		37		38		39		40	
41		42		43		44		45	
46		47		48		49		50	
51		52		53		54		55	
56		57		58		59		60	
61		62		63		64		65	
66		67		68		69		70	
71		72		73		74		75	
Total Wood		Total Fire		Total Earth		Total Metal		Total Water	

Appendix

FIVE ELEMENT TYPE
AND ACUPUNCTURE

Acupuncture has been mentioned at various times throughout this book and some of you may be wondering about the relationship between Five Element constitutional types and acupuncture treatment.

There are a number of different styles of acupuncture used to treat patients. This Five Element style of acupuncture is taught in a number of acupuncture colleges in Great Britain, Europe and the United States.

Practitioners using this treatment diagnose each patient's type (or Causative Factor as many acupuncturists call it) by observing the patient's facial colour, voice tone, emotion and odour. Having made the diagnosis they will also assess many of the characteristics of the 'type' which are discussed in this book. The changes gained from treatment are a crucial way of confirming the diagnosis. Improvements brought about by this kind of treatment should create shifts on many different levels and affect the patient's overall well-being.

Treatment is carried out by treating acupuncture points which are mainly sited along the energy pathways (or meridians) associated with the patient's main Elemental type. For example, an Earth type will be treated along the pathways of energy connected with the Stomach and Spleen, the two organs of the Earth Element. Likewise a Water type will be treated mainly on the Kidney and Bladder, the two organs of the Water Element.

This Five Element style of acupuncture is aimed at treating the whole person rather than the symptoms. In consequence patients often find that they feel much better inside as a result of treatment. Patients may also notice that some of their extremes of behaviour resulting from their type become less pronounced. Many of their presenting symptoms may also disappear.

Sometimes a patient's symptoms are not connected with their type. In this case other Elements or Organs need to be treated alongside the 'Causative Factor' so that the patient can be holistically healed. In this respect we, the authors, strongly believe that Five Element acupuncture should be integrated with the Yin-Yang style of treatment associated with what is commonly called Traditional Chinese Medicine (TCM).

The teaching of TCM includes the theory of Yin and Yang, the Substances (Qi, Blood, Essence, Body Fluids and Shen) and Pathogenic Factors (Wind, Cold, Damp, Heat, Dryness, Blood Stagnation and Phlegm). Practitioners who are trained in these two styles can holistically treat a wide range of patients. We also suggest that treatment can be greatly enhanced if used in conjunction with many of the exercises in this book. The use of these exercises will support patients so that they can gain greater insight into themselves as they grow and develop.

Here are the comments that two patients, Lorna and Jean, made to us about the results of treatment.

Lorna, an Earth type, said:

I went to treatment because I was very depressed. The doctor had suggested that I take anti-depressants but I wanted to get well naturally. I was very tearful at the time and not my usual bubbly self, in fact I felt really sorry for myself. The treatment put me back on an even keel and I now feel much more balanced inside and able to get on with my life once more.

Jean who is a Fire type told us:

I went for treatment with long-standing insomnia which was caused by feeling very anxious. I also used to fluctuate emotionally. Sometimes I'd feel really well then other times quite low. My practitioner and I have worked together and although it's taken a while for me to get better it has helped me tremendously. I can now sleep through the night and feel more stable in myself. I'm very grateful for what acupuncture has done.

Some of you may have found that you didn't recognize your type but are still curious about it. Others may have used the exercises but want to experience more. In this case you may wish to have treatment with an acupuncturist trained to diagnose and treat patients on their constitutional type. Not every acupuncturist is trained to treat this way. For more information, however, please ring or write to the British Acupuncture Council. You will find their address in the useful addresses section of this book.

BIBLIOGRAPHY

Books on Chinese Medicine and Chinese Language

Eckman, Peter, 1996: *In the Footsteps of the Yellow Emperor*; Cypress Book Company, San Francisco.

Hicks, Angela, 1996: *The Principles of Chinese Medicine*; Thorsons, London. This is a popular book which surveys Chinese medicine generally and the various treatment modalities.

Hicks, Angela, 1997: *The Principles of Acupuncture*; Thorsons, London. This is a popular book which surveys Chinese medicine generally and acupuncture treatment specifically.

Hicks, Angela, 1998: *The 5 Laws for Healthy Living*; Thorsons, London. This is a popular book which distils several thousand years of Chinese wisdom as to how to maintain your health through proper diet, regulation of the emotions, appropriate work, exercise and rest, protection from the environment and respecting our constitutions.

Hicks, John, 1997: *The Principles of Chinese Herbal Medicine*; Thorsons, London. This is a popular book which surveys Chinese medicine generally and Chinese herbal medicine specifically.

Larre, Claude, Schatz, Jean and Rochat de la Vallee, Elizabeth, 1986: *Survey of Traditional Chinese Medicine*; Institut Ricci, Paris, and Traditional Acupuncture Institute, Columbia, Maryland.

Maciocia, Giovanni, 1989: *The Foundations of Chinese Medicine*; Churchill Livingstone, Edinburgh. This is a textbook for students of Chinese medicine.

Maoshing Ni (trans), 1995: *The Yellow Emperor's Classic of Medicine*; Shambala,

Boston and London. This is one of the easier to read translations of the Nei Jing.

Mole, Peter, 1992: *Acupuncture, Energy Balancing for Body, Mind and Spirit*; Element Books, Dorset. This is a popular book which surveys Chinese medicine generally and acupuncture treatment specifically.

Koo, Linda Chih-ling, 1982: *Nourishment of Life*; The Commercial Press, Hong Kong.

Larre, Claude and Rochat de la Vallee, Elisabeth (trans), 1987: *The Secret Treatise of the Spiritual Orchid*; Monkey Press, Cambridge.

Weiger, L, 1965: *Chinese Characters*; Dover Publications, New York.

Books Relating to the Exercises or Emotions

Andreas, Connirae, 1994: *The Aligned Self* — audio-cassettes; NLP Comprehensive, Boulder, CO.

Andreas, Steve, 1991: *The Forgiveness Pattern* — audio-cassette; NLP Comprehensive, Boulder, CO.

Andreas, Connirae and Andreas, Steve, 1989: *Heart of the Mind*; Real People Press, Moab, Utah. This is a very useful account of the applications of NLP to a variety of emotional problems. It is both popular and useful.

Andreas, Steve and Faulkner, Charles, 1996: *NLP The New Technology of Achievement*; Nicholas Brealey, London. This is a popular book which runs through 43 exercises designed to create a context for and integrate your ambitions and actions to achieve them.

Bandler, Richard, 1985: *Using Your Brain — For a Change*; Real People Press, Moab, Utah. This is a book with a variety of useful, mind-changing exercises. It is the best description of the significance of how we represent things to ourselves in our minds.

Beck, Aaron T, 1976 and 1989: *Cognitive Therapy and the Emotional Disorders*; Penguin Books, London.

Beck, Aaron T, 1988: *Love is Never Enough*; Penguin Books, London.

Burns, David D, 1980: *Feeling Good*; Avon Books, New York. This is the best popular account of 'rational emotive therapy' which is one style of cognitive therapy.

Cornell, Ann Weiser, 1996: *The Power of Focusing*; New Harbinger Publications, Oakland, California.

Dilts, Robert B, 1994: *Strategies of Genius, Volume 1*; Meta Publications, Capitola, California.

Gendlin, Eugene T, 1978: *Focusing*; Bantam Book, New York.

Goleman, Daniel: 1995: *Emotional Intelligence*; Bloomsbury Publishing, London. This book outlines the concept of an emotional rather than an intellectual intelligence and argues the case from a Western point of view for emotional balance being a major contribution to health.

Hendrix, Harville, 1990: *Getting the Love You Want*; Harper Perennial, New York. This is a useful book if you are in a relationship and would like to improve the quality of love you are giving and getting. It requires you to work together and on your own and is recommended.

James, Oliver, 1997: *Britain on the Couch*; Century, London.

McDermott, Ian and O'Connor, Joseph, 1996a: *Principles of NLP*; Thorsons, London. This is a popular book and an excellent introduction to NLP.

McDermott, Ian and O'Connor, Joseph, 1996b: *NLP and Health*; Thorsons, London. This is a popular and readable discussion of the issue of health from an NLP point of view. There is a useful discussion of being in rapport with oneself as a foundation of health.

Ornstein, Robert and Sobel, David, 1989: *Healthy Pleasures*; Addison-Wesley, New York.

O'Hanlon Hudson, Patricia and Hudson O'Hanlon, William, 1991: *Rewriting Love Stories*; WW Norton and Company, New York and London. This book is from the therapists' point of view, but anyone wishing to become more adept at relating can learn a lot.

Books Relating to Qigong

Cohen, Kenneth, 1997: *The Way of Qigong*; Bantam Books, London and New York.

Guori, Jia, 1988: *Qigong Essentials for Health Promotion*; China Reconstructs Press, Beijing.

Hill, Sandra, 1997: *Reclaiming the Wisdom of the Body*; Constable, London.

Kit, Wong Kiew, 1997: *Chi Kung For Health and Vitality*; Element Books, Dorset. For a Qigong beginner, this is one of the most practical, easy to read and inspiring book.

Li Ding, 1988: *Meridian Qigong*; Foreign Language Press, Beijing.

Lin Housheng and Luo Peiyu, 1994: *300 Questions on Qigong Exercises*; Guandong Science and Technology Press, Guangzhou, China.

Yang, Jwing-Ming, 1996 second edition: *Tai Chi Theory and Martial Power*; YMAA Publication Center, Jamaica Plain, MA, USA.

Zhang, Mingwu and Sun, Xingyuan compilers, 1985: *Chinese Qigong Therapy*; Shandong Science and Technology Press, Jinan, China.

Zhizhong, Bian, 1987: *Daoist Health Preservation Exercises*; China Reconstructs Press, Beijing.

Biographies

Castle, Barbara, 1987: *Sylvia and Christabel Pankhurst*; Penguin Books, Harmondsworth, Middlesex, England. A book which describes the lives of Wood type Christabel Pankhurst and her sister Sylvia.

Greenstein, George, 1998: *Portraits of Discovery*; John Wiley and Sons, Inc, New York. Chapter 6 of this book is about Metal type Richard Feynman, 'All genius and all Buffoon'.

Kavanagh, David, 1998: *A Political Biography*; Oxford University Press, Oxford, England. This covers all the major figures in world politics including John F Kennedy.

Reeves, Thomas C, editor, 1990: *John F Kennedy*; Robert Krieger Publishing Co, Florida. Twenty-five essays written by different authors covering every aspect of Water type John F Kennedy's life.

Reeves, Thomas C, 1991: *A Life of John F Kennedy*; Bloomsbury Publishing Ltd, London. An investigation into the character of John F Kennedy.

Spoto, Donald, 1994: *Marilyn Monroe, The Biography*; Arrow Books, 1994, London. A fascinating biography of the every aspect of the life of Fire type Marilyn Monroe.

Various authors, 1998: *Biographical Dictionary of Women*; Penguin Books, London. Covers many famous women from all over the world, including Earth type Diana, Princess of Wales, Fire type Marilyn Monroe and Wood type Christabel Pankhurst.

USEFUL ADDRESSES

If you wish to find out more about any Chinese medicine treatments or to buy specialist Chinese medicine books you can contact the societies listed below.

UK

Acupuncture

British Acupuncture Council, Park House, 206 Latimer Road, London W10 2RE. Telephone: 0181 964 0222.

Qigong

Shen Hongxun Buqi Institute, c/o Sofie-Ann Bracke, 28 Brookfield Mansions, 5 Highgate West Hill, London N6 6AT. Telephone: 0181 347 9862.
Zhi Xing Wang and Wu Zhendi, Flat 3, 15 Dawson Place, London W2. Telephone: 0171 229 7187.

Neuro-Linguistic Programming

The Association of Neuro-Linguistic Programming (UK) Ltd, PO Box 78, Stourbridge, West Midlands, DY8 2YP. Telephone: 01384 443935; Fax: 01384 823448.

Specialist Books on Chinese Medicine

Acumedic 101–5 Camden High Street, London NW1 7JN. Telephone: 0171 388 6704.
East-West Herbs, Langston Priory Mews, Kingham, Oxfordshire OX7 6UP.
Telephone: 01608 658862; Fax: 01608 658816.
Harmony Medical Distribution, 629 High Road, Leytonstone, London E11 4PA.

If you wish to find out more information from the authors you can contact them at:
The College of Integrated Chinese Medicine, 19 Castle Street, Reading, Berkshire
RG1 7SB. Telephone: 0118 950 8880.

Australia

Acupuncture

Acupuncture Association of Victoria, 126 Union Road, Surrey Hills, Victoria 3127,
Australia. Telephone: 613 95322480.
Australia Acupuncture Ethics and Standards Organisation, PO Box 84, Merrylands,
New South Wales 2160, Australia. Telephone: 1800 025 334.
Australian Traditional Medicine Society, 120 Blaxland Road, Ryde, New South
Wales, 2112 Australia. Telephone: 809 6800.

Qigong

Qigong Association of Australia, 458 White Horse Road, Surrey Hills, Victoria 3127.
Telephone: 03-836-6961.

New Zealand

Acupuncture

New Zealand Register of Acupuncture, PO Box 9950, Wellington 1, New Zealand.
Telephone: 04 801 6400.

Qigong

David Hood, 341 Centaurus Road, St Martins, Christchurch 2, New Zealand. Telephone/Fax: 03 337 2838.

USA

Acupuncture

Council of Colleges of Acupuncture and Oriental Medicine, 1424 16th Street NW, Suite 501, Washington DC 20036. Telephone: 202 265 3370.
National Accreditation Commission for Schools and Colleges of Acupuncture and Oriental Medicine, 1010 Wayne Avenue, Suite 1270, Silver Spring, MD 20910. Telephone: 301 608 9680; Fax: 301 608 9576.
National Acupuncture and Oriental Medicine Alliance, 1833 North 105th Street, Seattle, Washington DC 98133. Telephone: 206 524 3511.
National Commission for the Certification of Acupuncturists, 1424 16th Street, NW, Suite 501, Washington DC 20036. Telephone: 202 332 5794.

Qigong

China Advocates, 1635 Irving Street, San Francisco, CA 94122. Telephone: 415 665 4505.
Qigong Academy, 8103 Marlborough Ave, Cleveland OH 44129. Telephone: 216 8742 9628.
Qigong Human Life Research Foundation, PO Box 5327, Cleveland OH 44101. Telephone: 415 788 2227.
The Qigong Institute, East West Academy of Healing Arts, 450 Sutter Street, Suite 916, San Francisco, CA 94108. Telephone: 818 564 9751.
Qigong Resource Associates, 1755 Homet Road, Pasadena, California 94122. Telephone: 818 564 9751.

Neuro-Linguistic Programming

NLP Comprehensive, 2897 Valmont Road, Colorado, 80301. Tel: 800 233 1657.

Specialist books on Chinese medicine

Redwing Reviews, Redwing Book Company, 44 Linden Street, Brookline, Massachusetts 02146 USA. Telephone: 617 738 4664. Orders (USA) 800 873 3946; Fax: 617 738 4620.

CANADA

Acupuncture

The Canadian Acupuncture Foundation, Suite 302, 7321 Victoria Park Avenue, Markham, Ontario L3R 278 Canada.

Qigong

Master Shou-Yu Liang, Shou-Yu Liang Wushu Institute, 7951 No 4 Road, Richmond, BC, Canada V6Y 2T4. Telephone: 604 228 3604; 604 273 9648.

INDEX